Healthcare Strategies for Patients with Chronic Diseases in an Ageing Society

Healthcare Strategies for Patients with Chronic Diseases in an Ageing Society

Editor

Hidetaka Hamasaki

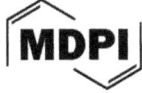

Basel • Beijing • Wuhan • Barcelona • Belgrade • Novi Sad • Cluj • Manchester

Editor
Hidetaka Hamasaki
Japan Medical Exercise Association
Yokohama
Japan

Editorial Office
MDPI AG
Grosspeteranlage 5
4052 Basel, Switzerland

This is a reprint of articles from the Special Issue published online in the open access journal *Healthcare* (ISSN 2227-9032) (available at: https://www.mdpi.com/journal/healthcare/special_issues/Ageing_Chronic_ehealth_mhealth).

For citation purposes, cite each article independently as indicated on the article page online and as indicated below:

Lastname, A.A.; Lastname, B.B. Article Title. *Journal Name* **Year**, *Volume Number*, Page Range.

ISBN 978-3-7258-2203-4 (Hbk)
ISBN 978-3-7258-2204-1 (PDF)
doi.org/10.3390/books978-3-7258-2204-1

© 2024 by the authors. Articles in this book are Open Access and distributed under the Creative Commons Attribution (CC BY) license. The book as a whole is distributed by MDPI under the terms and conditions of the Creative Commons Attribution-NonCommercial-NoDerivs (CC BY-NC-ND) license.

Contents

Mateja Lorber, Nataša Mlinar Reljić, Barbara Kegl, Zvonka Fekonja, Gregor Štiglic, Adam Davey and Sergej Kmetec
Person-Centred Care: A Support Strategy for Managing Non-Communicable Diseases
Reprinted from: *Healthcare* **2024**, *12*, 526, doi:10.3390/healthcare12050526 1

Cassie Doyle, Eunjeong Ko, Hector Lemus, Fang-Chi Hsu, John P. Pierce and Tianying Wu
Living Alone, Physical Health, and Mortality in Breast Cancer Survivors: A Prospective Observational Cohort Study
Reprinted from: *Healthcare* **2023**, *11*, 2379, doi:10.3390/healthcare11172379 14

Kyoko Hanari, Sandra Y. Moody, Takehiro Sugiyama and Nanako Tamiya
Preferred Place of End-of-Life Care Based on Clinical Scenario: A Cross-Sectional Study of a General Japanese Population
Reprinted from: *Healthcare* **2023**, *11*, 406, doi:10.3390/healthcare11030406 28

Jaime Barrio-Cortes, Almudena Castaño-Reguillo, Beatriz Benito-Sánchez, María Teresa Beca-Martínez and Cayetana Ruiz-Zaldibar
Utilization of Primary Healthcare Services in Patients with Multimorbidity According to Their Risk Level by Adjusted Morbidity Groups: A Cross-Sectional Study in Chamartín District (Madrid)
Reprinted from: *Healthcare* **2024**, *12*, 270, doi:10.3390/healthcare12020270 39

Linhong Chen and Xiaocang Xu
Poverty Reduction Effects of Medical Insurance on Middle-Aged and Elderly Families under the Goal of Common Prosperity in China
Reprinted from: *Healthcare* **2023**, *11*, 477, doi:10.3390/healthcare11040477 51

Thin Nyein Nyein Aung, Thaworn Lorga, Saiyud Moolphate, Yuka Koyanagi, Chaisiri Angkurawaranon, Siripen Supakankunti, et al.
Towards Cultural Adequacy of Experience-Based Design: A Qualitative Evaluation of Community-Integrated Intermediary Care to Enhance the Family-Based Long-Term Care for Thai Older Adults
Reprinted from: *Healthcare* **2023**, *11*, 2217, doi:10.3390/healthcare11152217 63

Rodrigo Cesar León Hernández, Jorge Luis Arriaga Martínez, Martha Arely Hernández Del Angel, Isabel Peñarrieta de Córdova, Virginia Solís Solís and María Elena Velásquez Salinas
Outcomes of a Self-Management Program for People with Non-Communicable Diseases in the Context of COVID-19
Reprinted from: *Healthcare* **2024**, *12*, 1668, doi:10.3390/healthcare12161668 76

Łukasz Goździewicz, Sławomir Tobis, Michał Chojnicki, Katarzyna Wieczorowska-Tobis and Agnieszka Neumann-Podczaska
The Value of the COVID-19 Yorkshire Rehabilitation Scale in the Assessment of Post-COVID among Residents of Long-Term Care Facilities
Reprinted from: *Healthcare* **2024**, *12*, 333, doi:10.3390/healthcare12030333 86

Matthew J. Wichrowski and Monica Moscovici
Horticultural Therapy for Individuals Coping with Dementia: Practice Recommendations Informed by Related Non-Pharmacological Interventions
Reprinted from: *Healthcare* **2024**, *12*, 832, doi:10.3390/healthcare12080832 97

Naima Z. Farhane-Medina, Rosario Castillo-Mayén, Bárbara Luque, Sebastián J. Rubio, Tamara Gutiérrez-Domingo, Esther Cuadrado, et al.
A Brief mHealth-Based Psychological Intervention in Emotion Regulation to Promote Positive Subjective Well-Being in Cardiovascular Disease Patients: A Non-Randomized Controlled Trial
Reprinted from: *Healthcare* **2022**, *10*, 1640, doi:10.3390/healthcare10091640 . . . . **111**

Hidetaka Hamasaki
Patient Satisfaction with Telemedicine in Adults with Diabetes: A Systematic Review
Reprinted from: *Healthcare* **2022**, *10*, 1677, doi:10.3390/healthcare10091677 . . . . **126**

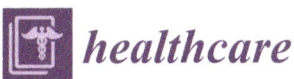

Article

Person-Centred Care: A Support Strategy for Managing Non-Communicable Diseases

Mateja Lorber [1,*], Nataša Mlinar Reljić [1], Barbara Kegl [1], Zvonka Fekonja [1], Gregor Štiglic [1], Adam Davey [2] and Sergej Kmetec [1,3]

1 Faculty of Health Sciences, University of Maribor, 2000 Maribor, Slovenia; natasa.mlinar@um.si (N.M.R.); barbara.kegl@um.si (B.K.); zvonka.fekonja@um.si (Z.F.); gregor.stiglic@um.si (G.Š.); sergej.kmetec1@um.si (S.K.)
2 College of Health Sciences, University of Delaware, Newark, DE 19716, USA; davey@udel.edu
3 Permanent Working Group of Palliative Care, Nurses and Midwives Association of Slovenia, 1000 Ljubljana, Slovenia
* Correspondence: mateja.lorber@um.si

Abstract: Background: Over the last decade, the inadequacy and unsustainability of current healthcare services for managing long-term co-morbid and multi-morbid diseases have become evident. Methods: This study, involving 426 adults with at least one non-communicable disease in Slovenia, aimed to explore the link between quality of life, life satisfaction, person-centred care, and non-communicable disease management. Results: Results indicated generally positive perceptions of quality of life, general health, and life satisfaction of individuals with non-communicable diseases. Participants assessed their physical health as the highest of the four quality of life domains, followed by the environment, social relations, and psychological health. Significant differences occurred in life satisfaction, general health, quality of life, and person-centred care for managing non-communicable diseases. But, there were no significant differences in person-centred care according to the living environment. The study revealed a positive association between person-centred care and effective non-communicable disease management, which is also positively associated with quality of life, general health, and life satisfaction. Conclusions: Person-centred care is currently the most compassionate and scientific practice conceived, representing a high ethical standard. However, implementing this approach in healthcare systems requires a cohesive national strategy led by capable individuals to foster stakeholder collaboration. Such an approach is crucial to address the deficiencies of existing healthcare services and ensure person-centred care sustainability in non-communicable disease management.

Keywords: person-centred care; non-communicable disease; quality of life; life satisfaction

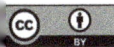

1. Introduction

Also referred to as chronic diseases, non-communicable diseases (e.g., cardiovascular diseases, cancers, chronic respiratory diseases, diabetes and others) typically persist for extended periods and arise from genetic, physiological, environmental, and behavioural influences. Annually, non-communicable diseases are responsible for 41 million deaths, which accounts for 74% of global fatalities, according to the World Health Organization [1]. The prevalence of non-communicable diseases escalates with age. Although the discourse on non-communicable diseases is predominantly centred on prevention, control, and the socio-economic factors influencing health, it is crucial to note that the overall impact of non-communicable diseases is also shaped by the demographic composition and age distribution of a country's population [2]. Non-communicable diseases present severe health risks for individuals, families, and communities and pose a potential threat to the capacity of healthcare systems. Given the significant socio-economic costs of non-communicable diseases, their prevention and control have become a crucial development goal for the

21st century [3]. It is also important to note that the quality of extended life—whether in good health or with illness—is vital for health system planners. They must comprehend the healthcare ramifications of an ageing population that could potentially experience long-term illnesses and complex multimorbidity [4]. Age is the primary determinant of risk for non-communicable diseases, as evidenced by studies conducted by Niccoli and Partridge [5] and Hou et al. [6]. However, the extent of age-related decline varies significantly among individuals, as noted by Elliott et al. [7] and Tuttle et al. [8]. It is noteworthy that a substantial proportion of the adult population, approximately half, grapples with one or more non-communicable diseases [5].

Consequently, individuals facing such conditions must confront many day-to-day challenges encompassing diverse symptoms, complications, loss of independence, and the self-management of non-communicable diseases. Additionally, it is pertinent to highlight that psychological distress experienced in the context of non-communicable diseases is linked to a decline in self-assessed health [9], a diminution in disease self-management, and adherence to lifestyle recommendations [10,11]. On a global scale, non-communicable diseases significantly impact numerous individuals' overall well-being and quality of life, exacerbated by rapid and unstructured urban development, the widespread adoption of detrimental habits, and an ageing population [12].

Distressing symptoms, such as fatigue, difficulties with sleep, weakness, and social seclusion, among others that arise from non-communicable illnesses, significantly diminish the well-being of individuals [13,14]. Individuals suffering from non-communicable diseases are frequently left to their own devices, necessitating substantial effort and time from themselves and their family members to make disease management decisions [15,16]. The provision of individualised care assumes a critical role in managing non-communicable diseases [17].

Person-centred care embodies a comprehensive and integrated methodology that esteems each individual as a distinct entity, encompassing their unique needs and values. This strategic approach customises care to address the specific non-communicable disease and the individual's condition, offering comprehensive care that attends to their physical, psychological, spiritual, and social requirements [17,18]. There is a lot of evidence that person-centred care is an effective therapeutic intervention for different patient outcomes [19–23]. In their rapid literature review, Cano et al. [22] discovered that implementing per-son-centred care models to foster self-care empowerment in long-term care resulted in multidimensional health-related outcomes. These outcomes have implications not only at the individual level but also at institutional and societal levels [22]. The development of self-awareness and the motivation for change can be fostered through personality assessments that acknowledge the intricate psychobiological makeup of human personality. The process of personality transformation is contingent on the interplay between an individual's physical, mental, and spiritual facets [23]. Person-centred care enhances individuals' quality of life and satisfaction and alleviates emotional strain on family members.

Moreover, this approach mitigates depression [24]. The primary objective of person-centred care is to uphold and enhance the quality of life for patients, their family members, and caregivers. Cultivating a sense of shared responsibility and collaborative decision-making in providing this type of care is crucial. A comprehensive body of literature, comprising 23,000 studies, has investigated the concept of person-centred care, either as a primary focus or as an integral component within broader research inquiries. Within this extensive collection, a meticulous review has discerned 921 studies specifically dedicated to exploring person-centred care. Among these, 503 studies directly employed methodologies tailored to measure the application of person-centred care, while 418 studies delved into associated aspects of this care paradigm. Methodological frameworks used within these studies encompassed a variety of approaches, including cross-sectional analyses (59%), qualitative methods such as interviews or focus groups (10%), observational techniques (6%), multi-methodological approaches (5%), and other diverse methodologies (8%) (de Silva, 2014). Furthermore, these investigations were geographically widespread, spanning regions such as the United Kingdom, Europe, North America, and other global territories [25].

Additionally, person-centred care is correlated with an improved quality of life and heightened satisfaction with care [26,27]. The person-centred approach underscores the humanisation of healthcare [26,28]. Berghout et al. [29] discovered that healthcare professionals also report positive experiences when delivering person-centred care.

Healthcare professionals' inadequate knowledge often impedes the implementation of person-centred care in the healthcare sector, creates a disregard for the person-centred approach, and highlights their inability to adapt to the individual's health condition. These obstacles can decrease individuals' quality of life and satisfaction, potentially leading to social isolation, despair, and self-identity loss [30,31].

Until now, the analysis of existing studies indicates a scarcity of research encompassing satisfaction with life, overall health, and the practice of person-centred care among individuals with non-communicable diseases. As a result, we aim to investigate the association between general health, life satisfaction, person-centred care, and the management of non-communicable diseases among adults with at least one non-communicable disease.

2. Materials and Methods

2.1. Design

The study used a quantitative cross-sectional methodology, using a validated survey instrument to gather data on various aspects, including overall health, life satisfaction, person-centred care, and disease management from individuals with non-communicable diseases. The study results' credibility was assured through strict adherence to the STROBE (Strengthening the Reporting of Observational Studies in Epidemiology) checklist [32].

2.2. Setting and Sample

This study used convenience sampling to recruit adult participants from the northeastern region of Slovenia. The sample selection was based on inclusion criteria: adult participants with at least one non-communicable disease. Conversely, the exclusion criteria encompassed participants younger than 18 (not adults) and those not diagnosed with a non-communicable disease. Following the Cochran formula [33] and considering the number of adults suffering from chronic disease (n = 433.230, recognising that this number is subject to constant fluctuations due to newly diagnosed diseases), our estimation revealed that the necessary sample size should consist of 384 participants. Out of the 640 questionnaires that were distributed, 439 were returned, resulting in a response rate of 69%. Following this, 13 questionnaires were excluded due to a non-completion rate of 50%, ultimately leading to a final sample size of 426 participants.

2.3. Study Tools/Instruments

Participants in this study completed a self-report questionnaire, including the World Health Organization Quality of Life-Bref version (WHOQOL-BREF) [34], the Satisfaction with Life Scale (SWLS) [35], and the Person-centred Practice Inventory for Service Users (PCPI-SU) [36], as well as questions about their demographics, such as physical activity, managing a non-communicable disease, income, social interaction, and support of loved ones.

The assessment of participants' quality of life was completed by utilising the WHOQOL-BREF [34], a questionnaire consisting of 26 items. This instrument encompasses four domains: physical health (7 items), psychological health (6 items), social relationships (3 items), and environment (8 items). Additionally, supplementary items are included to measure general health (1 item) and overall quality of life (1 item). Each item was evaluated by respondents using a 5-point Likert scale, where higher scores indicate an improved quality of life. The scores for each domain were calculated by summing the item scores within that specific domain and subsequently transformed to a 0–100 scale linearly. A score of 0 signifies the lowest possible health state, while a score of 100 indicates the highest possible health state within the respective domain.

Participants answered the question about managing non-communicable diseases on a four-point scale (very good to very poor).

The SWLS [35] questionnaire evaluated the participants' life satisfaction and consisted of five items. Respondents expressed their agreement or disagreement with each item using a 7-point scale, ranging from 7 (strongly agree) to 1 (strongly disagree). Possible scores range from 5 to 35, with predefined cut-offs categorising satisfaction levels as Extremely satisfied (31–35), Satisfied (26–30), Slightly satisfied (21–25), Neutral (20), Slightly dissatisfied (15–19), Dissatisfied (10–14), and Extremely dissatisfied (5–9).

The PCPI-SU [36], a 20-item questionnaire, aimed to capture individuals' perceptions of preserving person-centred care. This instrument encompasses five domains: working with the Person's Believe and Values (4 items), Sharing Decision-making (5 items), Engaging Authentically (4 items), Being Sympathetically Present (3 items) and Working Holistically (3 items). Grounded in McCormack and McCance's concepts of person-centred care [28], each statement was rated on a 5-point Likert scale, spanning from 'strongly disagree' (1) to 'strongly agree' (5). Higher scores on this instrument denoted a more positive perception of preserving person-centred care.

2.4. Data Collection

Data were gathered between January and June 2023, with previous ethical approval. The research team personally distributed questionnaires to all eligible participants and explained the study's aims to them. The participants were requested to complete the instrument conveniently and return it to the researcher in a sealed envelope within seven days at an agreed place. Following data collection, the information was entered into the SPSS Statistic 25 software (SPSS Inc., Chicago, IL, USA).

2.5. Data Analysis

This study's statistical analysis used both descriptive and inferential statistics. For demographic data, descriptive statistics, such as frequency, percentages, and mean and standard deviation estimates, were used. Categorical variables were presented as frequencies and percentages. The Shapiro–Wilk test was utilised to assess the normality distribution of variables. The results of this test indicated a departure from the normal distribution of the data. Considering the non-normal distribution, differences between the groups were assessed using either the Kruskal–Wallis or Mann–Whitney U-test. The Spearman correlation coefficient explored the associations among general health, life satisfaction, person-centred care, and non-communicable disease management. The significance level for all analyses was set at less than 0.05 to establish statistical significance. Furthermore, the internal consistency and reliability of the WHOQOL-BREF [34], SWLS [35], and PCPI-SU [36] questionnaires were evaluated using Cronbach's α coefficient.

2.6. Ethical Considerations

Before conducting the study, formal approval was sought from the relevant ethical committee (Ref. No: 038/2022/5006-4/902; approval 29 September 2022). Additionally, we obtained permission to conduct the study from nursing homes, health centres, and individual participants. Stringent ethical protocols were followed, with participants being presented with a participant information sheet attached to the first page of the questionnaire, delineating the study's aim and providing all necessary information. Subsequently, written consent was obtained from each participant. In recognition of the non-invasive nature of the study and the absence of any risks or hazards to the participants, informed verbal consent was deemed appropriate. The ethical conduct of the study adheres strictly to the principles outlined in the Declaration of Helsinki [37] and incorporates the provisions of the Oviedo Convention [38]. This ethical framework ensures the protection of participants' rights and upholds the integrity of the research process.

3. Results

The survey involved 426 participants from the northeastern region of Slovenia. The calculated Cronbach's α coefficients were 0.897 for WHOQOL-BREF, 0.876 for SWLS, and 0.816 for PCPI-SU. These coefficients reflect a high internal consistency and reliability level, affirming that the instruments consistently measure the intended constructs accurately and precisely. The demographics of the participants are presented in Table 1.

Table 1. Participant characteristics.

Variables	Descriptive Statistics Total (n = 426)
Gender %(n)	
Male	34.7 (148)
Female	65.3 (278)
Age (Year; M ± SD)	56.3 ± 17.6
Relationship Status %(n)	
Single	14.6 (62)
Married	41.8 (178)
Divorced	7 (30)
Cohabitation	24.6 (105)
Widowed	12 (51)
Education %(n)	
Elementary education	9.2 (39)
Secondary Education	51.9 (221)
HE (Bachelor)	30 (128)
HE (Master or Doctoral)	8.9 (38)
No. of NCD %(n)	
One	57.7 (246)
Two to three	40.1 (171)
Four or more	2.1 (09)
Managing NCD %(n)	
Very poor	7.5 (32)
Poor	9.2 (39)
Good	75.4 (321)
Very good	8.0 (34)

Note: n—Sample size; %—Percent of participants; M—Mean; SD—Standard deviation; HE—Higher Education; NCD—non-communicable disease.

A total of 426 patients with at least one non-communicable disease participated in the study. Among them, 65% were female, while 35% were male. The participants comprised 20% of individuals residing in nursing homes and 80% of community-dwelling adults with at least one non-communicable disease. The average age of the participants was 56.32 years (SD = 17.57). A substantial portion (42%) were married, and 25% cohabited. More than half (52%) of the participants had attained at least a secondary level of education, and a similar proportion (58%) reported having one non-communicable disease (Table 1).

From Table 2 we can see that according to the WHO-QOL-BREF, participants assessed as the highest physical health (M = 65.31; SD = 14.9; 95%; IC = 63.89–66.74), followed by the environment (M = 62.99; SD = 15.1; 95%; IC = 61.15–64.41); social relations (M = 59.49; SD = 19.5; 95%; IC = 57.71–61.25) and psychological health (M = 54.37; SD = 10.0; 95%; IC = 53.45–55.21). The highest value for person-centred care was the person's beliefs and values (M = 3.41; SD = 0.93; 95%; IC = 3.32–3.50), followed by the role of working holistically (M = 3.31; SD = 0.86; 95%; IC = 3.22–3.39), being sympathetically present (M = 3.30; SD = 0.87; 95%; IC = 3.22–3.38), sharing decision-making (M = 3.30; SD = 0.89;

95%; IC = 3.21–3.39) and engaging authentically (M = 3.29; SD = 0.86; 95%; IC = 3.21–3.37). The participant's quality of life score was 3.77 (SD = 0.72; 95%; IC = 3.70–3.85) and general health was 3.40 (SD = 1.01; 95%; IC = 3.31–3.50). Participants' life satisfaction averaged 24.23 (SD = 5.9; 95%; IC = 23.67–24.80).

Table 2. Descriptive data for general health, quality of life, life satisfaction, managing non-communicable disease and person-centred care.

Variables	M ± SD	Min–Max	Me ± IQR
General Health	3.40 ± 1.01	1–5	4.0 ± 1.0
Quality of life	3.77 ± 0.72	1–5	4.0 ± 1.0
Life satisfaction	24.23 ± 5.9	5–35	25.0 ± 9.0
Person-centred care	3.32 ± 0.83	1–5	3.18 ± 1.0
Person's believe and values	3.41 ± 0.93	1–5	3.25 ± 1.0
Sharing decision-making	3.30 ± 0.89	1–5	3.0 ± 1.0
Engaging authentically	3.29 ± 0.86	1–5	3.0 ± 1.0
Being sympathetically present	3.30 ± 0.87	1–5	3.3 ± 1.0
Working holistically	3.31 ± 0.86	1–5	3.25 ± 1.0
WHOQOL-BREF	60.54 ± 14.87	16.25–95.81	59.88 ± 17.5
Physical health	65.31 ± 14.9	10.75–100	64.5 ± 18.0
Psychological health	54.37 ± 10.0	12.5–83.25	54.0 ± 8.0
Social relationships	59.49 ± 19.5	16.75–100	58.5 ± 25.0
Environment	62.99 ± 15.1	25–100	62.5 ± 19.0
Managing NCD's	2.16 ± 0.67	1–4	2.0 ± 0

Note: M—Mean; SD—Standard deviation; Me—Median; IQR—Interquartile range; NCD—non-communicable disease.

As shown in Table 3, data indicate a significant difference in life satisfaction ($H(4) = 26.836$; $p < 0.001$), general health ($H(4) = 53.343$; $p < 0.001$), quality of life ($H(4) = 38.717$; $p < 0.001$) and person-centred care ($H(4) = 19.330$; $p < 0.001$) according to relationship status. There is a significant difference in life satisfaction ($H(3) = 22.590$; $p < 0.001$), general health ($H(3) = 23.174$; $p < 0.001$) and quality of life ($H(3) = 36.689$; $p < 0.001$) according to educational level. A significant difference was found in the quality of life according to the number of non-communicable diseases ($H(1) = 10.431$; $p < 0.001$) and frequency of physical activity ($H(4) = 27.186$; $p < 0.001$). Significant differences were found in life satisfaction ($H(3) = 18.128$; $p < 0.001$), general health ($H(3) = 45.364$; $p < 0.001$), quality of life ($H(3) = 33.386$; $p < 0.001$) and person-centred care ($H(3) = 11.622$; $p = 0.009$) according to the managing non-communicable disease.

Table 3. Demographic variables and their relationship with life satisfaction, satisfaction with health, quality of life and person-centred care.

Variables	Total (n = 426)	Life Satisfaction M ± SD (Me ± IQR)	General Health M ± SD (Me ± IQR)	Quality of Life M ± SD (Me ± IQR)	Person-Centred Care M ± SD (Me ± IQR)
Gender % (n)	—	U = 18,861.5 p = 0.156	U = 19,940.0 p = 0.582	U = 19,455.0 p = 0.277	U = 19,183.5 p = 0.248
Male	34.7 (148)	24.86 ± 5.49 (27.0 ± 7.0)	3.44 ± 0.97 (4.0 ± 1.0)	3.83 ± 0.69 (4.0 ± 1.0)	3.40 ± 0.81 (3.35 ± 1.0)
Female	65.3 (278)	23.89 ± 6.08 (24 ± 9.0)	3.38 ± 1.04 (4.0 ± 1.0)	3.74 ± 0.74 (4.0 ± 1.0)	3.29 ± 0.83 (3.11 ± 0.96)

Table 3. Cont.

Variables	Total (n = 426)	Life Satisfaction M ± SD (Me ± IQR)	General Health M ± SD (Me ± IQR)	Quality of Life M ± SD (Me ± IQR)	Person-Centred Care M ± SD (Me ± IQR)
Age (year) (M ± SD)	56.3 ± 17.6	$r_s = -0.243$ * $p < 0.001$	$r_s = -0.331$ * $p < 0.001$	$r_s = -0.350$ * $p < 0.001$	$r_s = 0.199$ * $p < 0.001$
Relationship Status % (n)	—	$H(4) = 26.836$ * $p < 0.001$	$H(4) = 53.343$ * $p < 0.001$	$H(4) = 38.717$ * $p < 0.001$	$H(4) = 19.330$ * $p < 0.001$
Single	14.6 (62)	23.53 ± 5.45 (24.0 ± 9.0)	3.69 ± 1.06 (4.0 ± 1.0)	3.77 ± 0.80 (4.0 ± 1.0)	3.02 ± 0.66 (3.0 ± 0.74)
Married	41.8 (178)	25.24 ± 5.54 (27.0 ± 8.0)	3.56 ± 0.96 (4.0 ± 1.0)	3.83 ± 0.71 (4.0 ± 1.0)	3.38 ± 0.94 (3.74 ± 1.0)
Divorced	7 (30)	23.13 ± 4.38 (23.0 ± 7.5)	2.70 ± 1.18 (3.0 ± 1.0)	3.80 ± 0.41 (4.0 ± 1.0)	3.39 ± 0.63 (3.26 ± 0.94)
Cohabitation	24.6 (105)	24.79 ± 5.74 (27.0 ± 9.0)	3.50 ± 0.92 (4.0 ± 0.0)	3.95 ± 0.59 (4.0 ± 1.0)	3.30 ± 0.73 (3.0 ± 0.65)
Widowed	12 (51)	21.04 ± 6.23 (22.0 ± 5.0)	2.73 ± 0.75 (3.0 ± 1.0)	3.20 ± 0.80 (3.0 ± 1.0)	3.49 ± 0.81 (3.42 ± 1.16)
Education % (n)	—	$H(3) = 22.590$ * $p < 0.001$	$H(3) = 23.174$ * $p < 0.001$	$H(3) = 36.689$ * $p < 0.001$	$H(3) = 3.719$ * $p = 0.293$
Elementary education	9.2 (39)	21.36 ± 7.08 (21.0 ± 11.0)	2.87 ± 1.22 (3.0 ± 1.0)	3.54 ± 0.97 (4.0 ± 1.0)	3.47 ± 0.74 (3.55 ± 1.03)
Secondary Education	51.9 (221)	23.68 ± 5.79 (24.0 ± 8.0)	3.34 ± 0.97 (3.0 ± 1.0)	3.62 ± 0.72 (4.0 ± 1.0)	3.32 ± 0.85 (3.20 ± 1.0)
HE (Bachelor)	30 (128)	27.27 ± 5.56 (27.0 ± 9.57)	3.70 ± 0.77 (4.0 ± 1.0)	4.04 ± 0.57 (4.0 ± 0.0)	3.29 ± 0.85 (3.0 ± 0.99)
HE (Master or Doctoral)	8.9 (38)	26.80 ± 4.63 (28.0 ± 6.0)	3.26 ± 1.41 (4.0 ± 1.0)	4.03 ± 0.59 (4.0 ± 0.0)	3.30 ± 0.66 (3.16 ± 0.65)
No. of NCD % (n)	—	$H(1) = 0.105$ $p = 0.745$	$H(1) = 0.276$ $p = 0.599$	$H(1) = 10.431$ * $p < 0.001$	$H(1) = 0.691$ $p = 0.496$
One	57.7 (246)	21.32 ± 5.97 (25.0 ± 8.0)	3.39 ± 1.02 (4.0 ± 1.0)	3.69 ± 0.76 (4.0 ± 1.0)	3.35 ± 0.91 (3.22 ± 1.0)
Two to three	40.1 (171)	24.26 ± 5.44 (25.0 ± 9.0)	3.44 ± 0.98 (4.0 ± 1.0)	3.92 ± 0.57 (4.0 ± 0.0)	3.31 ± 0.67 (3.10 ± 0.95)
Four or more	2.1 (09)	21.11 ± 10.83 (25 ± 20)	2.89 ± 1.36 (2.0 ± 2.0)	3.44 ± 1.51 (3.0 ± 3.0)	3.00 ± 0.85 (3.0 ± 0.98)
Managing NCD % (n)	—	$H(3) = 18.125$ * $p < 0.001$	$H(3) = 45.364$ * $p < 0.001$	$H(3) = 33.386$ * $p < 0.001$	$H(3) = 11.622$ * $p = 0.009$
Very poor	7.5 (32)	25.94 ± 4.22 (27.0 ± 6.5)	2.81 ± 1.26 (3.0 ± 1.0)	3.88 ± 0.55 (4.0 ± 2.0)	3.49 ± 0.72 (3.42 ± 0.74)
Poor	9.2 (39)	20.56 ± 5.62 (22.0 ± 8.0)	2.64 ± 0.71 (3.0 ± 1.0)	3.15 ± 0.75 (3.0 ± 1.0)	3.21 ± 0.91 (3.0 ± 1.0)
Good	75.4 (321)	24.39 ± 6.01 26.0 ± 9.0)	3.52 ± 0.96 (4.0 ± 1.0)	3.84 ± 0.69 (4.0 ± 0.0)	3.28 ± 0.82 (3.16 ± 0.96)
Very good	8.0 (34)	25.35 ± 5.01 (26.0 ± 7.5)	3.68 ± 1.01 (4.0 ± 1.0)	3.74 ± 0.83 (4.0 ± 1.0)	3.70 ± 0.79 (3.69 ± 1.30)
Contacts with loved ones % (n)	—	$H(3) = 4.779$ $p = 0.189$	$H(3) = 9.300$ * $p = 0.026$	$H(3) = 5.846$ $p = 0.119$	$H(3) = 3.455$ $p = 0.327$
Less than once/month	5.6 (24)	25.33 ± 3.75 24.0 ± 5.75)	2.88 ± 0.99 (3.0 ± 2.0)	3.83 ± 0.70 (4.0 ± 0.0)	3.56 ± 0.83 (3.73 ± 1.03)
Once/week to once/month	23.2 (99)	23.25 ± 5.74 (23.0 ± 9.0)	3.43 ± 0.94 (3.0 ± 1.0)	3.62 ± 0.78 (4.0 ± 1.0)	3.27 ± 0.71 (3.11 ± 0.96)
Few timed/week	31.9 (136)	24.04 ± 6.91 (26.0 ± 9.0)	3.50 ± 1.01 (4.0 ± 1.0)	3.83 ± 0.69 (4.0 ± 0.0)	3.29 ± 0.99 (3.05 ± 1.01)
Daily	39.2 (167)	24.81 ± 5.27 (25.0 ± 8.0)	3.81 ± 0.71 (4.0 ± 1.0)	3.81 ± 0.71 (4.0 ± 1.0)	3.35 ± 0.74 (3.20 ± 0.85)

Table 3. Cont.

Variables	Total (n = 426)	Life Satisfaction M ± SD (Me ± IQR)	General Health M ± SD (Me ± IQR)	Quality of Life M ± SD (Me ± IQR)	Person-Centred Care M ± SD (Me ± IQR)
Living environment	—	U = 10,202.5 * p < 0.001	U = 9566.0 * p < 0.001	U = 10,493.0 * p < 0.001	U = 13,612.0 * p < 0.001
Home environment	—	3.86 ± 0.67 (4 ± 1)	3.51 ± 0.98 (4 ± 1)	24.66 ± 6.05 (26 ± 8.25)	3.33 ± 0.84 (3.14 ± 1)
Nursing home	—	3.43 ± 0.81 (4 ± 1)	2.94 ± 1.03 (3 ± 2)	22.46 ± 4.88 (23 ± 6.75)	3.29 ± 0.76 (3.18 ± 0.95)
Physical activity % (n)	—	$H(4) = 6.827$ $p = 0.078$	$H(4) = 23.667$ * $p < 0.001$	$H(4) = 27.186$ * $p < 0.001$	$H(4) = 8.153$ * $p = 0.043$
Rarely	5.9 (25)	21.88 ± 9.03 (24.0 ± 15.5)	3.12 ± 1.33 (3.0 ± 2.0)	3.56 ± 0.92 (4.0 ± 1.0)	2.76 ± 0.97 (3.0 ± 0.75)
Very rare (1–4/month)	12 (51)	22.75 ± 5.09 (23.0 ± 7.0)	3.18 ± 0.84 (3.0 ± 1.0)	3.53 ± 0.67 (4.0 ± 1.0)	3.17 ± 0.88 (3.18 ± 1.13)
Rare (5–10/month)	41.3 (176)	24.24 ± 6.50 (24.5 ± 8.0)	3.00 ± 1.10 (3.0 ± 2.0)	3.59 ± 0.68 (4.0 ± 1.0)	3.36 ± 0.67 (3.11 ± 0.88)
Quite often (2.4/week)	24.4 (104)	24.44 ± 6.50 (26.0 ± 8.75)	3.60 ± 0.95 (4.0 ± 1.0)	3.92 ± 0.76 (4.0 ± 0.0)	3.36 ± 0.87 (3.18 ± 1.0)
Very often (5 or more/week)	16.4 (70)	25.60 ± 6.99 (27.0 ± 8.25)	3.77 ± 0.75 (4.0 ± 1.0)	3.94 ± 0.51 (4.0 ± 0.0)	3.49 ± 0.71 (3.50 ± 1.02)

Note: n—Sample size; %—Percent of participants; *—Statistical significance ($p < 0.05$); SD—Standard deviation; M—Mean; Me—Median; IQR—Interquartile range; HE—Higher Education; NCD—non-communicable disease; U—Mann–Whitney U test; H—Kruskal–Wallis test.

We also checked if any differences exist in the four domains of quality-of-life assessment. There were no differences according to gender, but there were significant differences in physical health ($H(4) = 15.909; p < 0.001$), psychological health ($H(4) = 23.420; p < 0.001$), social relations ($H(4) = 34.858; p < 0.001$) and environment ($H(4) = 25.124; p < 0.001$) according to relationship status. According to the number of non-communicable diseases, there were differences only in physical health ($H(1) = 7.410; p = 0.006$). The differences in physical health ($H(3) = 12.558, p = 0.006$), social relations ($H(3) = 16.317, p < 0.001$) and environment ($H(3) = 13.439, p = 0.004$) were found according to the managing non-communicable disease. Differences were found also in physical health ($H(4) = 47.395, p < 0.001$), psychological health ($H(4) = 17.451, p = 0.002$), social relations ($H(4) = 20.023, p < 0.001$), and environment ($H(4) = 36.920, p < 0.001$) according to the frequency of physical activity.

With Spearman correlation analysis it was found that the better management of non-communicable diseases is associated with physical health ($r_s = 0.118; p = 0.015$), psychological health ($r_s = 0.257; p < 0.001$), social relations ($r_s = 0.302, p < 0.001$), environment ($r_s = 0.292; p < 0.001$), contacts with loved ones ($r_s = 0.512; p < 0.001$), physical activity ($r_s = 0.267; p < 0.001$), economic status ($r_s = 0.133; p = 0.005$), and person-centred care ($r_s = 0.129; p = 0.009$). From the data, we also found that the level of managing non-communicable chronic disease is positively associated with quality of life ($r_s = 0.309; p < 0.001$) and general health ($r_s = 0.288; p < 0.001$). At the same time, quality of life ($r_s = 0.589; p < 0.001$) and general health ($r_s = 0.423; p < 0.001$) are positively associated with life satisfaction.

4. Discussion

Our study aimed to evaluate the management of non-communicable diseases, person-centred care, and their association with the quality of life and life satisfaction among adults afflicted with at least one non-communicable disease in Slovenia. The findings underscore the significance of person-centred care as an important variable in effectively managing non-communicable diseases and its influence on life satisfaction and overall quality of life. The data revealed significant differences across various domains, including life satisfaction, general health, quality of life, and person-centred care based on participants' relationship status. These findings suggest that individuals' relationship status is pivotal in determining their overall well-being and perception of care. Specifically, those in different relationship statuses may experience varying levels of satisfaction and health outcomes, highlighting the importance of considering relationship dynamics in healthcare interventions to enhance well-being.

Similarly, significant differences in life satisfaction, general health, and quality of life were observed based on participants' educational levels. This underscores the influence of educational attainment on individuals' perceptions of health and overall quality of life. Higher levels of education may be associated with better health outcomes and greater life satisfaction, possibly due to increased access to resources, knowledge, and opportunities for self-improvement. The study found significant differences in quality of life based on the number of non-communicable diseases and frequency of physical activity. This highlights the importance of disease management and regular physical activity in enhancing individuals' quality of life.

Moreover, it suggests that interventions targeting disease prevention and promoting physical activity could improve overall well-being among individuals. Significant differences were observed in various domains, including life satisfaction, general health, quality of life and person-centred care, based on how participants managed non-communicable diseases. This emphasises the need for personalised care approaches tailored to individuals' disease management strategies, as different approaches may impact their overall well-being and satisfaction with care differently. Examining the quality-of-life domains revealed further insights. While no differences were found according to gender, significant differences were observed in physical health, psychological health, social relations, and environment based on relationship status, number of non-communicable diseases, managing non-communicable diseases, and frequency of physical activity. These findings underscore the multidimensional nature of quality of life and highlight the importance of considering various factors when assessing individuals' well-being. Moreover, a weak, but consistent, magnitude-positive correlation was observed between enhanced non-communicable disease management and elevated quality of life, general health, life satisfaction, and favourable assessments in physical health, psychological health, social relations, environment, and person-centred care domains. These findings collectively contribute to a more comprehensive understanding of the intricate interplay between disease management, person-centred care, and individuals' health contending with non-communicable disease in the Slovenian context.

Most studies about person-centred care now focus on hospitalised patients [19,20,39] and older adults in long-term settings [21–23,40]. Our research included individuals with at least one non-communicable disease, regardless of the living environment, and we found that physical health, psychological health, social relationships, environment, contact with loved ones, and physical activities were positively associated with individuals' management of non-communicable disease. There were no significant differences in dimensions of person-centred care, not even in total, between participants according to the living environment, which is encouraging. Those living in the home environment and those living in nursing homes receive the same quality of person-centred care during the treatment of non-communicable diseases.

In the research, participants assessed their physical health as the highest of the four domains when they self-assessed their quality of life, followed by environment, social relations, and psychological health. In the psychological health domain, they barely achieved half the total value ($M = 54.4$; $SD = 10.0$). Compared with the research [41], which included 27 disease groups or health conditions and healthy people from 38 UK sites, they found that the environment was the highest assessed domain, followed by social relations and physical and psychological health. In that research, psychological health was assessed with a higher value ($M = 62.6$; $SD = 18$) than in our research. As in our study, Tseng et al. [41] also discovered a positive correlation between self-care and implementing person-centred care regarding psychological health. This suggests that introducing person-centred care models to encourage self-care empowerment achieves its goals. Tseng et al. [41] also highlighted that research has shown a direct link between general and self-rated health at the individual level.

Individuals already suffering from non-communicable diseases need to comprehend their identity, which enhances their understanding of how their lifestyle impacts their health, quality of life, and life satisfaction. Overall results for quality of life ($M = 3.77$; $SD = 0.7$), general health ($M = 3.40$; $SD = 1.0$), and life satisfaction ($M = 24.23$; $SD = 5.9$) were good. We found that 52% were very satisfied with their health, and 74% assessed their quality of life as good or very good. Our results are better compared to the results of Skevington et al. [42], who found that the quality of life and general health of participants in the UK was good and that 47% of the participants reported their quality of life as good and 37% were satisfied with their health.

Our research found that person-centred care is positively associated with the better management of non-communicable diseases and that managing non-communicable diseases is positively related to quality of life, general health, and life satisfaction. Other studies [19–23] showing that person-centred care is an effective therapeutic intervention for different patient outcomes support our results. In their rapid literature review, Cano et al. [22] discovered that implementing person-centred care models to foster self-care empowerment in long-term care resulted in multidimensional health-related outcomes with individual, institutional and societal implications.

The domains of person-centred care [43] typically first emerge in midlife; these elements are specifically for older adults with chronic conditions or functional impairments and support our results for adults with non-communicable diseases. According to our results, we should not overlook that it is next to person-centred care, and we have to point out the importance of the environment, social relations, and contacts with loved ones for the better management of non-communicable diseases and consequently better quality of life. We know that non-communicable disease necessitates extended supervision, monitoring, or care. To effectively address non-communicable diseases, healthcare employees must consider the individual's personal, family, social, political, cultural, and spiritual circumstances. Kogan et al. [43] noted that person-centred care is gaining prominence in all facets of healthcare, particularly in long-term residential care. This is especially true in light of the cultural evolution in caregiving for individuals with significant cognitive and other impairments, which includes various healthcare settings, long-term care, and social and community-based services for older adults.

Several limitations in this study warrant attention. Firstly, the study employed a cross-sectional design, which precludes the ability to draw causal conclusions. There is a scarcity of published studies comparing person-centred care and quality of life, mostly focusing on hospitalised patients and older adults in long-term settings. Secondly, a cross-sectional study can be subject to recall bias. Another potential limitation could be the sampling method used and its impact on the results. Given the predominance of one gender and location in the sample, the results cannot be generalised to the entire population.

Furthermore, the study relied on self-reported data, which could lead to social desirability bias, where respondents might overstate or understate their responses based on societal norms. No significant system failures were identified. The voluntary nature of participation in the study raises questions about whether the sample accurately represents the key characteristics of the population. Lastly, we could not account for all potential confounding factors that could influence the management of non-communicable disease and quality of life.

Despite the limitations, this study represents the initial strategies of healthcare for the improvement of management of non-communicable diseases, which consequently contribute to better quality of life and life satisfaction. This is particularly crucial because the number of older adults and the proportion of individuals with non-communicable diseases is rising. This presents a vital concern that, if not adequately assessed and managed by the healthcare system, it could adversely impact an individual's ability to fulfil their needs due to a decline in quality of life and life satisfaction. The primary objective of public health is to enhance quality of life, not just to promote independence in daily life. The help of community nurses largely addresses this goal. The necessity for person-centred strategies is evident in the traits of complex adaptive systems, which possess unique properties commonly found in numerous medical conditions. Within these complex adaptive systems, individuals with identical clinical characteristics can experience vastly different results, and conversely, those with varying clinical features may end up with the same outcome.

5. Conclusions

The growing trend of the life expectancy of the population, coupled with the prevalence of multiple non-communicable diseases and the heightened susceptibility of older adults, undeniably necessitates person-centred care as an essential strategy. This strategy emphasises the individual's active involvement in their healthcare treatment, encourages collaborative decision-making and mutual comprehension, and respects their values, preferences, and beliefs. Person-centred care diverts attention from the conventional biomedical approach, instead promoting the personal choice and independence of those who use health services. This strategy has proven to be an essential avenue for improving primary care, with older adults being key focuses of person-centred practice because they are more likely to have their care needs met compared to younger individuals.

Author Contributions: Conceptualisation: M.L., N.M.R., B.K., A.D., S.K. and Z.F.; Data curation, M.L., N.M.R., B.K. and Z.F. and S.K.; Formal analysis, M.L., S.K., G.Š. and Z.F.; Methodology, M.L., S.K., B.K. and G.Š.; Supervision, M.L., S.K., N.M.R. and A.D.; Writing—original draft, M.L. and S.K.; and Writing—review and editing, M.L., N.M.R., B.K., Z.F., G.Š., A.D. and S.K. All authors have read and agreed to the published version of the manuscript.

Funding: A study reported in this publication was supported by the Slovenian Research Agency (BI-US/22-24-096) and the National Cancer Institute of the National Institutes of Health under Award Number R01CA194178. The content is solely the responsibility of the authors and does not necessarily represent the official views of the National Institutes of Health.

Institutional Review Board Statement: The study was conducted in accordance with the Declaration of Helsinki and approved by the Ethics Committee of the University of Maribor, Faculty of Health Sciences (Ref. No: 038/2022/5006-4/902; approval 29 September 2022).

Informed Consent Statement: Participants were informed of their option to withdraw before submitting the questionnaire. By responding to the survey, participants indicated their consent to participate in the study. Written approval was obtained from all institutions where the questionnaire was administered. The patient(s) has obtained written informed consent to publish this paper.

Data Availability Statement: Additional data from this study are not publicly available to maintain participants' anonymity.

Acknowledgments: The authors thank all participants for participating in the study.

Conflicts of Interest: The authors declare no conflicts of interest.

References

1. World Health Organization. Noncommunicable Diseases: Key Facts. Available online: https://www.who.int/news-room/fact-sheets/detail/noncommunicable-diseases (accessed on 27 December 2023).
2. de Lacy-Vawdon, C.; Livingstone, C. Defining the commercial determinants of health: A systematic review. *BMC Publ. Health* **2020**, *20*, 1022. [CrossRef]
3. World Health Organization: Noncommunicable Diseases. Available online: https://www.who.int/health-topics/noncommunicable-diseases#tab=tab_1 (accessed on 27 December 2023).
4. Moffat, K.; Mercer, S.W. Challenges of managing people with multimorbidity in today's healthcare systems. *BMC Fam. Pract.* **2015**, *16*, 129. [CrossRef] [PubMed]
5. Niccoli, T.; Partridge, L. Ageing as a risk factor for disease. *Curr. Biol.* **2012**, *22*, R741–R752. [CrossRef] [PubMed]

6. Hou, Y.; Dan, X.; Babbar, M.; Wei, Y.; Hasselbalch, S.G.; Croteau, D.L.; Bohr, V.A. Ageing as a risk factor for neurodegenerative disease. *Nat. Rev. Neurol.* **2019**, *15*, 565–581. [CrossRef]
7. Elliott, M.L.; Caspi, A.; Houts, R.M.; Ambler, A.; Broadbent, J.M.; Hancox, R.J.; Harrington, H.; Hogan, S.; Keenan, R.; Knodt, A.; et al. Disparities in the pace of biological aging among midlife adults of the same chronological age have implications for future frailty risk and policy. *Nat. Aging* **2021**, *1*, 295–308. [CrossRef] [PubMed]
8. Tuttle, C.S.L.; Waaijer, M.E.C.; Slee-Valentijn, M.S.; Stijnen, T.; Westendorp, R.; Maier, A.B. Cellular senescence and chronological age in various human tissues: A systematic review and meta-analysis. *Aging Cell* **2020**, *19*, e13083. [CrossRef]
9. Hajat, C.; Stein, E. The global burden of multiple chronic conditions: A narrative review. *Prev. Med. Rep.* **2018**, *12*, 284–293. [CrossRef]
10. DiMatteo, M.R.; Lepper, H.S.; Croghan, T.W. Depression is a risk factor for noncompliance with medical treatment: Meta-analysis of the effects of anxiety and depression on patient adherence. *Arch. Intern. Med.* **2000**, *160*, 2101–2107. [CrossRef]
11. Prince, M.; Patel, V.; Saxena, S.; Maj, M.; Maselko, J.; Phillips, M.R.; Rahman, A. No health without mental health. *Lancet* **2007**, *370*, 859–877. [CrossRef]
12. World Health Organization. *Global Action Plan for the Prevention and Control of Noncommunicable Diseases 2013–2020*; World Health Organization: Geneva, Switzerland, 2013.
13. Dionne-Odom, J.N.; Azuero, A.; Lyons, K.D.; Hull, J.G.; Tosteson, T.; Li, Z.; Li, Z.; Frost, J.; Dragnev, K.H.; Akyar, I.; et al. Benefits of Early Versus Delayed Palliative Care to Informal Family Caregivers of Patients with Advanced Cancer: Outcomes From the ENABLE III Randomized Controlled Trial. *J. Clin. Oncol.* **2015**, *33*, 1446–1452. [CrossRef]
14. Sandsdalen, T.; Grøndahl, V.A.; Hov, R.; Høye, S.; Rystedt, I.; Wilde-Larsson, B. Patients' perceptions of palliative care quality in hospice inpatient care, hospice day care, palliative units in nursing homes, and home care: A cross-sectional study. *BMC Palliat. Care* **2016**, *15*, 79. [CrossRef]
15. Ahluwalia, S.C.; Chen, C.; Raaen, L.; Motala, A.; Walling, A.M.; Chamberlin, M.; O'Hanlon, C.; Larkin, J.; Lorenz, K.; Akinniranye, O.; et al. A Systematic Review in Support of the National Consensus Project Clinical Practice Guidelines for Quality Palliative Care, Fourth Edition. *J. Pain Symptom Manag.* **2018**, *56*, 831–870. [CrossRef]
16. Bausewein, C.; Simon, S.T.; Pralong, A.; Radbruch, L.; Nauck, F.; Voltz, R. Palliative Care of Adult Patients with Cancer. *Dtsch. Arztebl. Int.* **2015**, *112*, 863–870. [CrossRef]
17. Kmetec, S.; Fekonja, Z.; Kolarič, J.; Reljić, N.M.; McCormack, B.; Sigurðardóttir, Á.K.; Lorber, M. Components for providing person-centred palliative healthcare: An umbrella review. *Int. J. Nurs. Stud.* **2022**, *125*, 104111. [CrossRef] [PubMed]
18. McCormack, B.; Dewing, J. International Community of Practice for Person-centred Practice: Position statement on person-centredness in health and social care. *Int. Pract. Dev. J.* **2019**, *9*, 1–7. [CrossRef]
19. Klancnik Gruden, M.; Turk, E.; McCormack, B.; Stiglic, G. Impact of Person-Centered Interventions on Patient Outcomes in Acute Care Settings: A Systematic Review. *J. Nurs. Care Qual.* **2021**, *36*, E14–E21. [CrossRef] [PubMed]
20. Tay, F.H.E.; Thompson, C.L.; Nieh, C.M.; Nieh, C.C.; Koh, H.M.; Tan, J.J.C.; Yap, P.L.K. Person-centered care for older people with dementia in the acute hospital. *Alzheimers Dement.* **2018**, *4*, 19–27. [CrossRef] [PubMed]
21. Abbott, K.M.; Klumpp, R.; Leser, K.A.; Straker, J.K.; Gannod, G.C.; Van Haitsma, K. Delivering Person-Centered Care: Important Preferences for Recipients of Long-term Services and Supports. *J. Am. Med. Dir. Assoc.* **2018**, *19*, 169–173. [CrossRef] [PubMed]
22. Cano, F.; Alves, E.; João, A.; Oliveira, H.; Pinho, L.G.; Fonseca, C. A rapid literature review on the health-related outcomes of long-term person-centred care models in adults with chronic illness. *Front. Public. Health* **2023**, *11*, 1213816. [CrossRef] [PubMed]
23. Downey, J.; Bloxham, S.; Jane, B.; Layden, J.D.; Vaughan, S. Person-Centered Health Promotion: Learning from 10 Years of Practice within Long Term Conditions. *Healthcare* **2021**, *9*, 439. [CrossRef] [PubMed]
24. Kim, S.; Tak, S.H. Validity and Reliability of the Korean Version of Person-Centered Practice Inventory-Staff for Nurses. *J. Korean Acad. Nurs.* **2021**, *51*, 363–379. [CrossRef] [PubMed]
25. de Silva, D. *Helping Measure Person-Centred Care: A Review of Evidence about Commonly Used Approaches and Tools Used to Help Measure Person-Centred Care*; The Health Foundation: London, UK, 2014.
26. Phelan, A.; McCormack, B.; Dewing, J.; Brown, D.; Cardiff, S.; Cook, N.; Dickson, C.; Kmetec, S.; Lorber, M.; Magowan, R.; et al. Critical Review of Literature Review of Developments in Person-Centred Healthcare. *Int. Pract. Dev. J.* **2020**, *10*, 4. [CrossRef]
27. Teeling, S.; Dewing, J.; Baldie, D. A Discussion of the Synergy and Divergence between Lean Six Sigma and Person-Centred Improvement Sciences. *Int. J. Res. Nurs.* **2020**, *11*, 10–23. [CrossRef]
28. McCance, T.; McCormack, B. The person-centred practice framework. In *Fundamentals of Person-Centred Healthcare Practice*; McCormack, B., McCance, T., Bulley, C., Brown, D., McMillan, A., Martin, S., Eds.; Wiley-Blackwell: Oxford, UK, 2021; pp. 23–32.
29. Berghout, M.; van Exel, J.; Leensvaart, L.; Cramm, J.M. Healthcare professionals' views on patient-centered care in hospitals. *BMC Health Serv. Res.* **2015**, *15*, 385. [CrossRef] [PubMed]
30. Berntsen, G.; Høyem, A.; Lettrem, I.; Ruland, C.; Rumpsfeld, M.; Gammon, D. A person-centered integrated care quality framework, based on a qualitative study of patients' evaluation of care in light of chronic care ideals. *BMC Health Serv. Res.* **2018**, *18*, 479. [CrossRef] [PubMed]
31. Lavoie, M.; Blondeau, D.; Martineau, I. The integration of a person-centered approach in palliative care. *Palliat. Support. Care* **2013**, *11*, 453–464. [CrossRef]

32. von Elm, E.; Altman, D.G.; Egger, M.; Pocock, S.J.; Gøtzsche, P.C.; Vandenbroucke, J.P. The Strengthening the Reporting of Observational Studies in Epidemiology (STROBE) statement: Guidelines for reporting observational studies. *J. Clin. Epidemiol.* **2008**, *61*, 344–349. [CrossRef]
33. Cochran, W.G. *Sampling Techniques*; John Wiley & Sons: New York, NY, USA, 1977.
34. World Health Organization. WHOQOL-BREF. Available online: https://www.who.int/tools/whoqol/whoqol-bref (accessed on 27 December 2023).
35. Diener, E.; Emmons, R.A.; Larsen, R.J.; Griffin, S. The Satisfaction with Life Scale. *J. Pers. Assess.* **1985**, *49*, 71–75. [CrossRef]
36. McCance, T.e.a. The Person-Centred Practice Inventory—Service User. Available online: https://www.cpcpr.org/resources (accessed on 27 December 2023).
37. Idänpään-Heikkilä, J.E. Ethical principles for the guidance of physicians in medical research: The Declaration of Helsinki. *Bull. World Health Organ.* **2001**, *79*, 279. [PubMed]
38. Conseil de l'Europe. *Convention for the Protection of Human Rights and Dignity of the Human Being with Regard to the Application of Biology and Medicine: Convention on Human Rights and Biomedicine*; Conseil de l'Europe: Strasbourg, France, 1997.
39. Al-Sahli, B.; Eldali, A.; Aljuaid, M.; Al-Surimi, K. Person-Centered Care in a Tertiary Hospital Through Patient's Eyes: A Cross-Sectional Study. *Patient Prefer. Adherence* **2021**, *15*, 761–773. [CrossRef] [PubMed]
40. Li, J.; Porock, D. Resident outcomes of person-centered care in long-term care: A narrative review of interventional research. *Int. J. Nurs. Stud.* **2014**, *51*, 1395–1415. [CrossRef] [PubMed]
41. Tseng, M.Y.; Yang, C.T.; Liang, J.; Huang, H.L.; Kuo, L.M.; Wu, C.C.; Cheng, H.S.; Chen, C.Y.; Hsu, Y.H.; Lee, P.C.; et al. A family care model for older persons with hip-fracture and cognitive impairment: A randomised controlled trial. *Int. J. Nurs. Stud.* **2021**, *120*, 103995. [CrossRef] [PubMed]
42. Skevington, S.M.; McCrate, F.M. Expecting a good quality of life in health: Assessing people with diverse diseases and conditions using the WHOQOL-BREF. *Health Expect.* **2012**, *15*, 49–62. [CrossRef]
43. Kogan, A.C.; Wilber, K.; Mosqueda, L. Person-Centered Care for Older Adults with Chronic Conditions and Functional Impairment: A Systematic Literature Review. *J. Am. Geriatr. Soc.* **2016**, *64*, e1–e7. [CrossRef] [PubMed]

Disclaimer/Publisher's Note: The statements, opinions and data contained in all publications are solely those of the individual author(s) and contributor(s) and not of MDPI and/or the editor(s). MDPI and/or the editor(s) disclaim responsibility for any injury to people or property resulting from any ideas, methods, instructions or products referred to in the content.

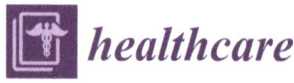

Article

Living Alone, Physical Health, and Mortality in Breast Cancer Survivors: A Prospective Observational Cohort Study

Cassie Doyle [1], Eunjeong Ko [2], Hector Lemus [1], Fang-Chi Hsu [3], John P. Pierce [4] and Tianying Wu [1,4,*]

1. Division of Epidemiology and Biostatistics, School of Public Health, San Diego State University, San Diego, CA 92182, USA; cdoyle3871@sdsu.edu (C.D.); hlemus@sdsu.edu (H.L.)
2. School of Social Work, San Diego State University, San Diego, CA 92182, USA; eko@sdsu.edu
3. Department of Biostatistics and Data Science, Division of Public Health Sciences, Wake Forest University School of Medicine, Winston-Salem, NC 27101, USA; fhsu@wakehealth.edu
4. Moores Cancer Center, School of Medicine, University of California, San Diego, CA 92037, USA; jppierce@ucsd.edu
* Correspondence: tianying.wu@sdsu.edu; Tel.: +1-(619)-594-0969

Abstract: Living alone, particularly for individuals with poor physical health, can increase the likelihood of mortality. This study aimed to explore the individual and joint associations of living alone and physical health with overall mortality among breast cancer survivors in the Women's Healthy Eating and Living (WHEL). We collected baseline, 12-month and 48-month data among 2869 women enrolled in the WHEL cohort. Living alone was assessed as a binary variable (Yes, No), while scores of physical health were measured using the RAND Short Form–36 survey (SF-36), which include four domains (physical function, role limitation, bodily pain, and general health perceptions) and an overall summary score of physical health. Cox proportional hazard models were used to evaluate associations. No significant association between living alone and mortality was observed. However, several physical health measures showed significant associations with mortality (p-values < 0.05). For physical function, the multivariable model showed a hazard ratio (HR) of 2.1 (95% CI = 1.02–4.23). Furthermore, the study examined the joint impact of living alone and physical health measures on overall mortality. Among women with better physical function, those living alone had a 3.6-fold higher risk of death (95% CI = 1.01–12.89) compared to those not living alone. Similar trends were observed for pain. However, regarding role limitation, the pattern differed. Breast cancer survivors living alone with worse role limitations had the highest mortality compared to those not living alone but with better role limitations (HR = 2.6, 95% CI = 1.11–5.95). Similar trends were observed for general health perceptions. Our findings highlight that living alone amplifies the risk of mortality among breast cancer survivors within specific health groups.

Keywords: living alone; physical health; mortality; breast cancer survivor; social isolation

1. Introduction

Breast cancer ranks as the second leading cause of cancer-related mortality among women in the United States [1]. Recent data from January 2022 indicates a population of over 3.8 million female breast cancer survivors in the country [2]. The American Cancer Society defines a breast cancer survivor as any individual who has ever received a cancer diagnosis, irrespective of their current stage of treatment [1].

Survivors of breast cancer have reported a range of physical health challenges during and after their treatment, including fatigue, pain, sleep disturbances, and gastrointestinal issues such as constipation [3]. In addition to these physical ailments, survivors also encounter emotional, psychological, and social concerns. These encompass apprehension regarding cancer metastasis or recurrence, feelings of depression, body image disturbances, changes in interpersonal relationships, and financial burdens [3]. These stressors can adversely impact the well-being and survival of women following a breast cancer diagnosis.

Citation: Doyle, C.; Ko, E.; Lemus, H.; Hsu, F.-C.; Pierce, J.P.; Wu, T. Living Alone, Physical Health, and Mortality in Breast Cancer Survivors: A Prospective Observational Cohort Study. *Healthcare* **2023**, *11*, 2379. https://doi.org/10.3390/healthcare11172379

Academic Editors: Hidetaka Hamasaki and Eiji Nakatani

Received: 5 July 2023
Revised: 16 August 2023
Accepted: 17 August 2023
Published: 24 August 2023

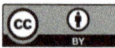

Copyright: © 2023 by the authors. Licensee MDPI, Basel, Switzerland. This article is an open access article distributed under the terms and conditions of the Creative Commons Attribution (CC BY) license (https://creativecommons.org/licenses/by/4.0/).

In a comprehensive advisory spanning 85 pages, Surgeon General Vivek Murthy, MD, MBA, released a declaration in May 2023, recognizing loneliness and isolation as significant public health epidemics within the United States [4]. Extensive research has consistently demonstrated a link between social isolation and unfavorable health behaviors, including suboptimal dietary choices, smoking, and physical inactivity [5–7]. Furthermore, individuals who experience loneliness and social isolation often face heightened challenges in coping with stress, trauma, adversity, anxiety, and depression [4]. Consequently, breast cancer survivors who also face social isolation are at an increased risk of diminished long-term survival [8,9].

Living alone can contribute to social isolation, as individuals who live by themselves may have limited opportunities for social interaction and companionship. In early 2021, an estimated 37 million adults in the United States aged 18 and older, comprising approximately 15% of the population, were residing alone [10]. These rates of solitary living have been consistently rising and are expected to continue on an upward trajectory [6,10]. While previous studies have investigated social isolation in the context of marital status, social interactions, church group involvement, and community organization membership, less is known specifically about the implications of living alone as an isolated measure among breast cancer survivors [9,11]. However, the existing research on the association between living alone and mortality among various cancer populations has produced limited and mixed findings [6,12–14].

Although prior investigations have established a relationship between physical health outcomes and mortality risk in cancer patients [15], no study, to our knowledge, has specifically examined the joint impacts of living alone and physical health on mortality among female breast cancer survivors. This research gap is noteworthy because the influence of living alone on mortality may be contingent upon other factors, such as an individual's physical health status.

Therefore, the objective of this study is to assess both the independent and combined associations of living alone and physical health with all-cause mortality among female breast cancer survivors in the United States. We will utilize longitudinal data from the Women's Healthy Eating and Living (WHEL) study to investigate this relationship.

2. Materials and Methods

2.1. Study Design and Population

This study utilizes data from a pre-existing prospective cohort derived from the WHEL study, which enrolled a total of 3088 female breast cancer survivors between 1995 and 2000, with an average follow-up period of 7.3 years [16]. The WHEL study was a randomized clinical trial supported by the National Institutes of Health (NIH), conducted at seven sites across California, Arizona, Texas, and Oregon [16]). Its primary objective was to investigate the potential benefits of intensive dietary intervention, emphasizing a rich intake of vegetables, fruit, and fiber while minimizing fat consumption, on reducing the incidence of subsequent breast cancer events and premature mortality in women with early-stage invasive breast cancer [16]. Participant recruitment for the study involved a multi-faceted approach, incorporating tumor registries, collaboration with community oncologists, and community outreach initiatives [16]. Detailed information regarding the inclusion and exclusion criteria can be found in the original publication of the WHEL study [16]. In summary, eligible participants were breast cancer survivors aged 18 to 70, with stage I ($\geq$1 cm), II, or IIIA breast cancer diagnosed within the previous four years, not currently scheduled for or undergoing chemotherapy, able to provide dietary data through 24-h food recalls, and exhibiting no evidence of recurrent disease, cancer recurrence, or new breast cancer [16]. Exclusion criteria encompassed pregnancy, the presence of life-threatening diseases or medical conditions, and the diagnosis of comorbidities requiring specific dietary regimens or contraindicating a high-fiber diet due to medication use [16]. Additionally, our study employed supplementary exclusion criteria targeting individuals with missing baseline data on living alone status and physical functioning scores, resulting in a final cohort comprising 2869 women. The data analysis was performed as an observational study rather than a clinical trial, given that the risk factors under examination in this cohort were not the original randomized interventions.

2.2. Assessment of Living Alone Status and Physical Health

Living alone status was evaluated as a dichotomous variable, categorizing participants as either living alone or not living alone at three time points: baseline, year 1, and year 4.

Physical health was assessed through the Medical Outcomes Study (MOS) 36-Item Short Form Health Survey (SF-36), a validated instrument developed by RAND in 1992, which specifically measures various aspects of physical health [17]. The SF-36 encompasses four physical health scales, namely physical functioning, role limitations due to physical health problems, bodily pain, and general health perceptions [17]. These scales have been rigorously validated and demonstrate a high level of reliability, with Cronbach's alpha coefficients ranging from 0.78 to 0.93 [17,18].

The physical functioning scale consists of ten items that assess an individual's ability to engage in moderate and vigorous physical activities, including tasks such as walking, climbing, bending, and lifting [17]. Role limitations due to physical health are evaluated through four items that examine the extent to which individuals experience limitations in work or other regular activities, such as difficulties in completing tasks or the need for frequent rest [17]. The bodily pain scale comprises two items that measure the degree to which pain interferes with daily activities, encompassing work and household tasks [17]. General health perceptions involve five items that inquire about individuals' overall assessment of their current health status [17].

Detailed scoring instructions for each scale can be accessed on RAND's website [19]. Each subscale of physical health is scored on a range from 0 to 100, with higher scores indicating better health. To determine the overall physical health score, the mean of the four physical health subscales was calculated [20].

2.3. Assessment of Study Outcome

The primary outcome of this investigation is total mortality. By the conclusion of the study in June 2006, the vital status of 95% of participants in the intervention group and 96% of those in the comparison group was established [21]. Participants who were lost to follow-up were considered censored at the date of their last contact. To determine mortality information, a confirmation interview was conducted with participants, and the medical records and/or death certificates were reviewed independently by two oncologists. Additionally, a search was performed on the National Death Index [16]. The Social Security Death Index (updated until 2009).

Survival analysis was performed by calculating the time from study entry to the occurrence of death. For participants without an event, the follow-up time was censored either at the time of the last documented contact with the study staff or at the completion of the study in June 2006 [16].

2.4. Assessments of Covariates

At baseline, standardized questionnaires were employed to gather information on participants' demographic, behavioral, and lifestyle characteristics. These characteristics, along with self-reported health status, encompassing comorbid conditions (e.g., cardiovascular conditions, digestive conditions, arthritis, osteoporosis) and medications such as blood sugar, cardiovascular, and gastrointestinal medications, were documented [16]. Relevant variables pertaining to the patient's medical records were also extracted, including their initial cancer diagnosis and treatment details [16]. Variables concerning cancer status and treatment encompassed hormone receptor status and the utilization of radiation or chemotherapy [16].

To evaluate physical activity levels, an adapted and validated Personal Habits Questionnaire from the Women's Health Initiative was employed [22]. Physical activity was quantified using metabolic equivalent tasks (METs), as employed in prior studies [23]. Additionally, social support was evaluated utilizing the 9-item MOS social support scale, which exhibited good internal consistency with a Cronbach's alpha of 0.75 [17].

2.5. Statistical Analyses

All data analyses were performed using SAS version 9.4 (SAS Institute, Cary, NC, USA). To assess the differences in baseline characteristics, we employed the χ^2 test for categorical variables and *t*-test and analysis of variance (ANOVA) for normally distributed continuous variables for both (a) living alone status, physical function score, role limitation score, pain score, general health score, and overall physical health score and (b) mortality status.

Living alone status was treated as a binary variable (Yes, No), while the physical function summary score ($\leq$Median, >Median) and all other physical health scores (<Median, $\geq$Median) were categorized into two groups for ease of interpretation. Repeated measures of living alone status and physical health scores at years 0, 1, and 4 were analyzed as time-varying covariates.

Cox proportional hazard models were utilized to examine the independent and joint associations of living alone and each subscale of physical health with all-cause mortality. Hazard ratios (HRs) and their corresponding 95% confidence intervals (CIs) were used to estimate these associations. We examined the joint associations by creating joint variables of living alone with each subscale of physical health. Each joint variable consisted of 4 groups of living arrangements and each individual physical health subscale. We first divided each physical health subscale into two categories using the median score as a cut-point. Then, we created the 4 joint groups to represent the interaction of physical function and living arrangements. The four groups include Physical function score > median combined with not living alone, physical function score > median combined with living alone, physical function score $\leq$ median combined with not living alone, and physical function score $\leq$ median combined with living alone. Analogous procedures were employed to generate all remaining joint variables. We included relevant covariates in our models.

Adjustments were made for the following covariates based on a priori assumptions: age at diagnosis (years), cancer stage (I, II, IIIA), chemotherapy (Yes, No), radiotherapy (Yes, No), hormone status (ER+/PR+, Other), ethnicity (White, Non-white), social support summary score (2–42, 42–67, 67–89, 89–100), body mass index (BMI) in kg/m^2 (Underweight, Healthy weight, Overweight, Obese), alcohol consumption in g (0, $\leq$0.14, 0.14–5.95, 5.95–16.17, >16.17), physical activity in METs/week ($\leq$225, 225–675, 675–1350, and >1350), smoking status (Never smoker, Past smoker with less than 15 pack years, Past smoker with 15 or more pack years, Current smoker), menopausal status (Premenopausal, Postmenopausal, Perimenopausal), and medical conditions requiring medications (None, 1, 2, 3 or more). Time-varying covariates included the social support summary score, BMI, alcohol intake, physical activity, and smoking status. Baseline data were used for the other covariates. As the main study was a randomized trial, we included group assignment (Intervention, Comparison) in the model to account for the possibility of intervention effects on other variables. The proportional hazards assumption was assessed and met for all Cox proportional hazard regression models.

3. Results

3.1. Baseline Characteristics

Table 1 presents the baseline characteristics of the 2869 women included in the study. Most participants were White (85.6%), with a mean age of 50.8 years at the time of diagnosis. A large proportion of these women did not live alone (83.8%) and were postmenopausal (79.7%). Approximately 56.3% of the participants had physical function scores equal to or lower than the median score of 90. Furthermore, a considerable number of women underwent chemotherapy (69.7%), and radiotherapy (61.4%), and 58.2% had no medical conditions requiring medications. Among the participants, 62.0% were classified as ER+/PR+, and 54.1% were never smokers. Nearly half of the participants had a healthy weight (42.1%), and approximately 31.4% reported no alcohol intake.

Table 1. Baseline characteristics of the WHEL study participants ($n = 2869$).

	Overall	Mortality Status		p-Value
		No ($n = 2581$)	Yes ($n = 288$)	
Live alone				0.016
No	2404 (83.8)	2177 (84.4)	227 (78.8)	
Yes	465 (16.2)	404 (15.7)	61 (21.2)	
Physical function score				0.0002
≤90	1615 (56.3)	1423 (55.1)	192 (66.7)	
>90	1254 (43.7)	1158 (44.8)	96 (33.3)	
Role limitation score				<0.0001
<100	1317 (45.9)	1150 (44.6)	167 (58.0)	
≥100	1550 (54.0)	1429 (55.4)	121 (42.0)	
Pain score				
<87.5	1433 (50.0)	1270 (49.2)	163 (56.6)	0.0027
≥87.5	1435 (50.0)	1310 (50.8)	125 (43.4)	
General health score				0.0025
<75	1322 (46.1)	1165 (45.1)	157 (54.5)	
≥75	1547 (53.9)	1416 (54.9)	131 (45.5)	
Overall physical health score				0.034
<43.125	2090 (72.9)	1865 (72.3)	225 (78.1)	
≥43.125	779 (27.2)	716 (27.7)	63 (21.9)	
Age at diagnosis (years)	50.8 ± 8.8	50.8 ± 8.7	51.4 ± 10.1	0.24
Randomization group				0.78
Intervention	1427 (49.7)	1286 (49.8)	141 (49.0)	
Comparison	1442 (50.3)	1295 (50.2)	147 (51.0)	
Cancer Stage				<0.0001
I	1107 (38.6)	1054 (40.8)	53 (18.4)	
II	1618 (56.4)	1422 (55.1)	196 (68.1)	
IIIA	144 (5.0)	105 (4.1)	39 (13.5)	
Chemotherapy				0.0016
Yes	1997 (69.7)	1773 (68.8)	224 (77.8)	
No	870 (30.4)	806 (31.3)	64 (22.2)	
Radiation therapy				0.89
Yes	1760 (61.4)	1582 (61.34)	178 (61.8)	
No	1105 (38.6)	995 (38.6)	110 (38.2)	
Hormone status				<0.0001
ER+/PR+	1778 (62.0)	1631 (63.2)	147 (51.0)	
Other	1091 (38.0)	950 (36.8)	141 (49.0)	
Ethnicity				0.18
White	2457 (85.6)	2218 (85.9)	239 (83.0)	
Non-white	412 (14.4)	363 (14.1)	49 (17.0)	
Social support summary score (quartile)				0.50
2–42	142 (5.0)	122 (4.7)	20 (6.9)	
42–67	522 (18.2)	475 (18.4)	47 (16.3)	
67–89	1126 (39.3)	1015 (39.3)	111 (38.5)	
89–100	1078 (37.6)	968 (37.5)	110 (38.2)	
BMI (kg/m^2)				0.0063
Underweight (0–18.5)	28 (1.0)	23 (0.9)	5 (1.7)	
Healthy weight (18.5–25)	1209 (42.1)	1108 (42.9)	101 (35.1)	
Overweight (25–30)	885 (30.9)	799 (31.0)	86 (29.9)	
Obese (≥30)	747 (26.0)	651 (25.2)	96 (33.3)	
Alcohol consumption (g)				0.13
0	902 (31.4)	799 (31.0)	103 (35.8)	
≤0.14	492 (17.2)	434 (16.8)	58 (20.1)	
0.14–5.95	709 (24.7)	646 (25.0)	63 (21.9)	
5.95–16.17	448 (15.6)	410 (15.9)	38 (13.2)	
>16.17	318 (11.1)	292 (11.3)	26 (9.0)	

Table 1. Cont.

	Overall	Mortality Status		p-Value
		No (n = 2581)	Yes (n = 288)	
Physical activity (METs/week)				0.0072
≤225	805 (28.1)	713 (27.6)	92 (31.9)	
225–675	710 (24.8)	625 (24.2)	85 (29.5)	
675–1350	715 (24.9)	648 (25.1)	67 (23.3)	
>1350	639 (22.3)	595 (23.1)	44 (15.3)	
Smoking status				<0.0001
Never smoker	1553 (54.1)	1409 (54.6)	144 (50.0)	
Past smoker with less than 15 pack years	750 (26.1)	692 (26.8)	58 (20.1)	
Past smoker with 15 or more pack years	421 (14.7)	357 (13.8)	64 (22.2)	
Current smoker	126 (4.4)	110 (4.3)	16 (5.6)	
Menopausal status				0.049
Premenopausal	313 (10.9)	271 (10.5)	42 (14.6)	
Postmenopausal	2283 (79.7)	2057 (79.8)	226 (78.5)	
Perimenopausal	269 (9.4)	249 (9.7)	20 (6.9)	
Tumor Size (centimeters)				<0.0001
≤2	1667 (58.3)	1563 (60.8)	104 (36.1)	
>2	1194 (41.7)	1010 (39.3)	184 (63.9)	
Medical conditions that require medications				0.036
None	1670 (58.2)	1507 (58.4)	163 (56.6)	
1	691 (24.1)	615 (23.8)	76 (26.4)	
2	349 (12.2)	324 (12.6)	25 (8.7)	
3 or more	159 (5.5)	135 (5.2)	24 (8.3)	

Categorical variables are presented as N, % (column %). Continuous variables are presented as mean ± SD. Abbreviations: ER = estrogen receptor; PR = progesterone receptor; BMI = body mass index; METs = metabolic equivalents. Bolded p-Values indicate statistical significance using a significance level (α) of 0.05.

Throughout the follow-up period, a total of 288 deaths occurred. Comparing women who experienced all-cause mortality to those without any deaths, we observed higher rates of living alone (21.2%), physical functioning scores below the median (66.7%), obesity based on BMI (33.3%), a history of smoking with 15 or more pack years (22.2%), and a higher likelihood of belonging to the lower two groups of physical activity, reporting less than 675 METs of physical activity per week (61.4%). The p-values for these comparisons were <0.05.

3.2. Baseline Characteristics Stratified by Physical Function Score and Living Arrangement

Table 2 presents the unadjusted bivariate associations between baseline characteristics and physical function scores, as well as living alone status. In comparison to women with better physical health based on their function scores, women with poorer health were more likely to be older, overweight, or obese, have lower social support scores (falling into the two lowest categories), report lower levels of physical activity (falling into the two lowest categories), and have one, two, or three or more medical conditions requiring medications. As indicated in Table 2, women who lived alone, in contrast to those who did not, were more likely to be older and have lower social support scores (falling into the three lowest categories). Additionally, women who lived alone were less likely to have never smoked and to have undergone chemotherapy. The p-values for these comparisons were <0.05.

Table 2. Bivariate associations of baseline characteristics with physical function scores and living arrangements among breast cancer survivors (n = 2869).

	Physical Function Score			Live Alone		
	>90	≤90	p-Value	No	Yes	p-Value
Age at diagnosis (years)	49.2 ± 8.8	52.1 ± 8.7	**<0.0001**	50.3 ± 8.8	53.7 ± 8.7	**<0.0001**
Randomization group			0.96			0.46
Intervention	623 (49.7)	804 (49.8)		1203 (50.0)	224 (48.2)	
Comparison	631 (50.3)	811 (50.2)		1201 (50.0)	241 (51.8)	
Cancer Stage			0.081			0.95
I	492 (39.2)	615 (38.1)		927 (38.6)	180 (38.7)	
II	712 (56.8)	906 (56.1)		1355 (56.4)	263 (56.6)	
IIIA	50 (4.0)	94 (5.8)		122 (5.1)	22 (4.7)	
Chemotherapy			0.48			**<0.0001**
Yes	882 (70.3)	1115 (69.1)		1718 (71.5)	279 (60.0)	
No	372 (29.7)	498 (30.9)		684 (28.5)	186 (40.0)	
Radiation therapy			0.85			0.60
Yes	771 (61.6)	989 (61.3)		1480 (61.6)	280 (60.3)	
No	480 (38.4)	625 (38.7)		921 (38.4)	184 (39.7)	
Hormone status			0.49			0.77
ER+/PR+	786 (62.7)	992 (61.4)		1487 (61.9)	291 (62.6)	
Other	468 (37.3)	623 (38.6)		917 (38.1)	174 (37.4)	
Social support summary score (Quartile)			**<0.0001**			**<0.0001**
2–42	37 (2.9)	105 (6.5)		86 (3.6)	56 (12.0)	
42–67	179 (14.2)	350 (21.5)		380 (15.7)	149 (32.0)	
67–89	498 (39.5)	635 (39.0)		949 (39.2)	184 (39.5)	
89–100	547 (43.4)	537 (33.0)		1007 (41.6)	77 (16.5)	
BMI (kg/m^2)			**<0.0001**			0.046
Underweight (0–18.5)	14 (1.1)	14 (0.9)		19 (0.8)	9 (1.9)	
Healthy weight (18.5–25)	695 (55.1)	514 (31.6)		1000 (41.3)	209 (44.9)	
Overweight (25–30)	378 (30.0)	507 (31.1)		754 (31.1)	131 (28.1)	
Obese (≥30)	167 (13.2)	580 (35.6)		631 (26.0)	116 (24.9)	
Alcohol consumption (g)			**<0.0001**			0.18
0	354 (28.1)	548 (33.7)		746 (30.8)	156 (33.5)	
≤0.14	183 (14.5)	329 (20.2)		432 (17.8)	80 (17.2)	
0.14–5.95	308 (24.4)	401 (24.6)		612 (25.3)	97 (20.8)	
5.95–16.17	236 (18.7)	212 (13.0)		376 (15.5)	72 (15.5)	
>16.17	180 (14.3)	138 (8.5)		257 (10.6)	61 (13.1)	
Physical activity (METs/week)			**<0.0001**			0.21
0–225	215 (17.1)	590 (36.2)		690 (28.5)	115 (24.7)	
225–675	286 (22.7)	424 (26.0)		587 (24.2)	123 (26.4)	
675–1350	349 (27.7)	366 (22.5)		589 (24.3)	126 (27.0)	
>1350	404 (32.0)	235 (14.4)		538 (22.2)	101 (21.7)	
Smoking status			0.15			**<0.0001**
Never smoker	693 (55.0)	860 (52.8)		1355 (55.9)	198 (42.5)	
Past smoker with less than 15 pack years	338 (26.8)	412 (25.3)		618 (25.5)	132 (28.3)	
Past smoker with 15 or more pack years	162 (12.9)	259 (15.9)		320 (13.2)	101 (21.7)	
Current smoker	54 (4.3)	72 (4.4)		95 (3.9)	31 (6.7)	
Menopausal status			**<0.0001**			**<0.0001**
Premenopausal	191 (15.3)	122 (7.6)		288 (12.0)	25 (5.4)	
Postmenopausal	951 (76.0)	1332 (82.6)		1884 (78.4)	399 (86.2)	
Medical conditions that require medications			**<0.0001**			0.15
None	875 (69.8)	795 (49.2)		1421 (59.1)	249 (53.6)	
1	267 (21.3)	424 (26.3)		569 (23.7)	122 (26.2)	
2	91 (7.3)	258 (16.0)		283 (11.8)	66 (14.2)	
3 or more	21 (1.7)	138 (8.5)		131 (5.5)	28 (6.0)	

Categorical variables are presented as N, % (column %). Continuous variables are presented as mean ± SD. Abbreviations: ER = estrogen receptor; PR = progesterone receptor; BMI = body mass index; METs = metabolic equivalents. Bolded p-Values indicate significance using a statistical significance level (α) of 0.05.

3.3. Independent Associations of Living Alone, Physical Function, and Other Physical Health Scores with Mortality

The associations of living alone, physical function, role limitation, pain, general health, and overall physical health with all-cause mortality are presented in Table 3. Age-adjusted and multivariable-adjusted analyses were conducted to assess these associations.

Table 3. Independent associations of living alone and each physical health measure with total mortality.

	Category	Age-Adjusted HR (95% CI)	Multivariable-Adjusted HR (95% CI)
Living alone	No	Ref	Ref
	Yes	1.3 (0.72–2.53)	1.4 (0.75–2.78)
Physical function	>90	Ref	Ref
	≤90	2.7 (1.36–5.19) *	2.1 (1.02–4.23) *
Role limitation	≥100	Ref	Ref
	<100	2.0 (1.16–3.59) *	1.8 (1.03–3.32) *
Pain	≥87.5	Ref	Ref
	<87.5	1.3 (0.77–2.28)	1.1 (0.63–1.97)
General health	≥75	Ref	Ref
	<75	2.6 (1.47–4.56) *	2.6 (1.41–4.67) *
Overall physical health	≥43.125	Ref	Ref
	<43.125	2.5 (1.20–5.10) *	1.9 (0.86–4.03)

* p-value < 0.05. The multivariable-adjusted model was adjusted for intervention group, age at diagnosis, BMI, cancer stage, estrogen and progesterone status, alcohol consumption, physical activity levels, social support, smoking status, radiotherapy, chemotherapy, menopausal status, and number of comorbidity medications.

No significant association between living alone and all-cause mortality was found. The age-adjusted hazard ratio (HR) for living alone was 1.3 (95% CI = 0.72–2.53), while the multivariable-adjusted HR was 1.4 (95% CI = 0.75–2.78).

A significant association was observed between physical function and all cause mortality (p-value < 0.05). In the age-adjusted model, women with lower physical function had a higher risk of death, with an HR of 2.7 (95% CI = 1.36–5.19). After adjusting for covariates in the multivariable model, the association remained significant but slightly attenuated, with an HR of 2.1 (95% CI = 1.02–4.23). Role limitation due to physical health issues was also significantly associated with all-cause mortality (p-value < 0.05). The age-adjusted HR for role limitation was 2.0 (95% CI = 1.16–3.59), and the multivariable-adjusted HR was 1.8 (95% CI = 1.03–3.32).

No significant association was found between pain and mortality. However, general health showed a significant association with all-cause mortality (p-value < 0.05), with an age-adjusted HR of 2.6 (95% CI = 1.47–4.56) and a multivariable-adjusted HR of 2.6 (95% CI = 1.41–4.67).

Regarding overall physical health, a significant association with mortality was observed in the age-adjusted model, with an HR of 2.5 (95% CI = 1.20–5.10). However, in the multivariable-adjusted model, the association was not statistically significant, with an HR of 1.9 (95% CI = 0.86–4.03).

3.4. Joint Associations of Physical Health and Living Alone with Mortality

The joint impacts of living alone and each subscale of physical health on all-cause mortality were examined. Table 4, Figures 1 and 2 present the results of these joint associations.

Table 4. Joint associations of living alone and each physical health measure with mortality.

		Living Alone	
		No HR (95% CI)	Yes HR (95% CI)
Physical function			
	>90	Ref	3.6 (1.01–12.89) *
	≤90	2.8 (1.20–6.61) *	2.7 (0.96–7.64)
Role limitation			
	≥100	Ref	0.9 (0.25–3.11)
	<100	1.6 (0.84–3.10)	2.6 (1.11–5.95) *
Pain			
	≥87.5	Ref	2.6 (1.05–6.55) *
	<87.5	1.5 (0.78–2.90)	1.2 (0.45–3.14)
General health			
	≥75	Ref	1.0 (0.33–3.24)
	<75	2.3 (1.16–4.48) *	4.0 (1.66–9.82) *
Overall physical health			
	≥43.125	Ref	1.6 (0.78–3.09)
	<43.125	2.2 (0.97–5.10)	1.1 (0.14–8.60)

* p-value < 0.05. The multivariable-adjusted model was adjusted for intervention group, age at diagnosis, BMI, cancer stage, estrogen and progesterone status, alcohol consumption, physical activity levels, social support, smoke years, radiotherapy, chemotherapy, menopausal status, and number of comorbidity medications.

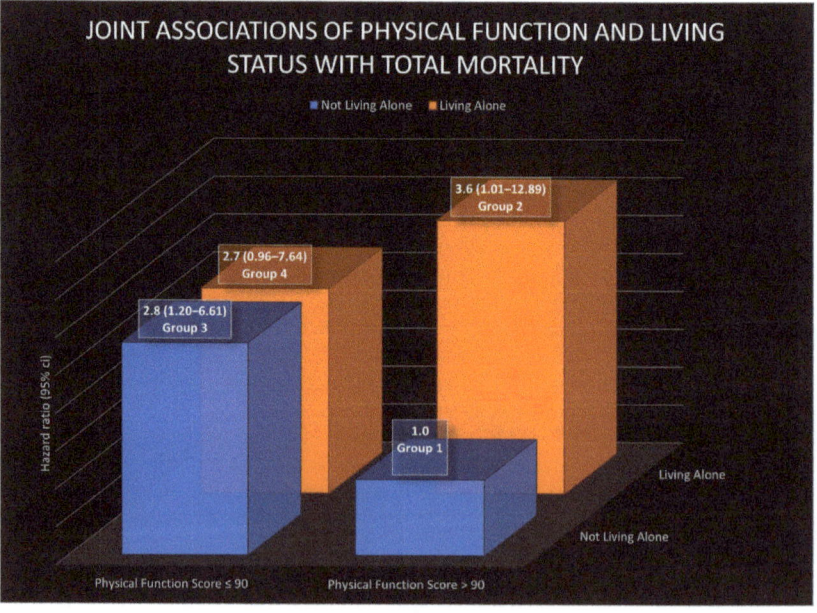

Figure 1. The hazard ratios in this chart were adjusted for intervention group, age at diagnosis, body mass index, cancer stage, estrogen and progesterone status, alcohol consumption, physical activity levels, social support, smoke years, radiotherapy, chemotherapy, menopausal status, and number of comorbidity medications.

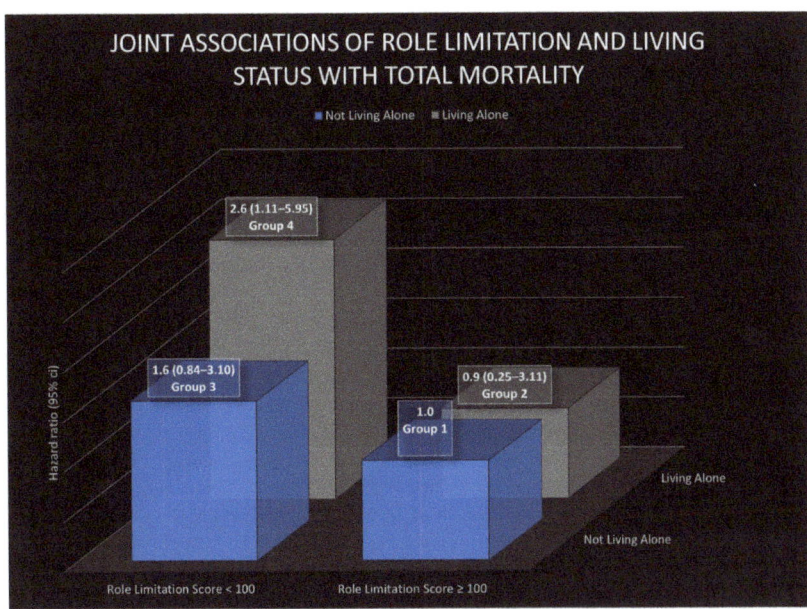

Figure 2. The hazard ratios in this chart were adjusted for intervention group, age at diagnosis, body mass index, cancer stage, estrogen and progesterone status, alcohol consumption, physical activity levels, social support, smoke years, radiotherapy, chemotherapy, menopausal status, and number of comorbidity medications.

As seen in Table 4 and Figure 1, among women with higher physical function, those who were living alone showed a significantly higher rate of death compared to women who were not living alone and had higher physical function scores (p-value < 0.05). The hazard ratio (HR) was 3.6 (95% CI = 1.01–12.98), indicating that women living alone with higher physical function had 3.6 times the risk of mortality compared to the reference group. In contrast, for individuals with lower physical function scores, the HRs were similar between women who lived alone and those who did not live alone, with HRs ranging from 2.7 to 2.8 and significant or marginally significant confidence intervals.

Furthermore, the joint associations of living alone with role limitation, pain, general health, and overall physical health on all-cause mortality were examined, as presented in Table 4. Similar trends were observed for the joint associations of pain with living alone, resembling the joint associations of physical function with living alone. However, for role limitation and general health, the trends of the joint associations differed somewhat. As seen in Table 4 and Figure 2, Group 4, which consisted of individuals living alone with lower levels of role limitation or general health, exhibited the highest mortality compared to the reference group (Group 1), with hazard ratios of 2.6 (95% CI = 1.11–5.95) for role limitation and 4.0 (95% CI = 1.66–9.82) for general health.

In contrast to other measures, the joint analysis of living alone and overall physical health revealed that living alone did not further increase the risk of mortality in either the groups with lower or higher scores of overall physical health.

Overall, these findings highlight the complex interplay between living alone and various aspects of physical health in relation to all-cause mortality.

4. Discussion

The results of our study revealed significant associations between several measures of physical health and an increased risk of total mortality. While living alone showed a positive association with total mortality, the independent association did not reach statistical significance. Additionally, we observed the joint associations between living alone and various physical measures in relation to mortality.

Regarding role limitation and general health, individuals who lived alone and had lower levels of role limitation or general health exhibited a greater risk of mortality compared to those who also lived alone but had higher levels of role limitation or better general health. Conversely, for physical function and pain, living alone significantly increased the risk of mortality among individuals with better physical function or better levels of pain. However, for these two measures, living alone did not further amplify the risk of mortality among individuals with worse levels of physical function or worse levels of pain.

Our finding regarding the significant association between physical health and higher mortality rates aligns with previous studies [8,15,24,25]. However, the association between living alone and total mortality did not reach statistical significance, possibly due to the relatively shorter follow-up time of 6 years in our study. The lack of a significant association between living alone and higher mortality rates has been reported in some studies, indicating that living alone is not the sole predictor of mortality in general and cancer-specific populations [6,12–14]. The estimated hazard ratio for the association between living alone and mortality in our study falls within the range of estimates reported by prior studies, which ranged from 0.93 to 1.81 [6,13,14].

It should be noted that living alone does not necessarily lead to mortality. However, it may contribute to individuals receiving limited instrumental support [9], which could explain why living alone, in conjunction with poor physical health, accelerates the risk of mortality, particularly concerning role limitation and general health measures. The reasons underlying the increased mortality risk associated with living alone in the high physical function and lower pain group but not in the low physical function or high pain group remain unclear. Nonetheless, it is essential to recognize that lower physical function itself is significantly associated with mortality, suggesting that the impact of living alone on mortality may be relatively small compared to the effect of physical function. This could elucidate why significant associations were not observed in the latter group, although the presence of measurement errors or residual confounding cannot be entirely ruled out. Nevertheless, our findings highlight that living alone amplifies the risk of mortality within specific physical health groups.

This analysis possesses several strengths. Notably, it employed a joint modeling approach to assess the simultaneous associations of living alone, physical functioning, and additional physical health measures with mortality. We utilized validated and standardized scales to measure quality of life, and serial measurements were employed to capture living alone and physical function over time. Moreover, our study encompassed a substantial sample size of women with early-stage breast cancer, with a follow-up period of 7.3 years, affording adequate statistical power to identify associations with mortality and control for potential confounding variables, including demographic and lifestyle factors. Furthermore, reported deaths were verified through death certificates, and vital status was confirmed using the National Death Registry.

A limitation of our study is that we utilized a single, well-validated, yet questionnaire-based measure (SF-36) instead of employing multiple objective measures. The reliance on self-reported responses for these measures introduces the potential for measurement errors influenced by bias. Although socioeconomic status adjustment was not feasible, we did control for social support within our study. Additionally, our sample predominantly consisted of White breast cancer survivors, limiting the generalizability of our findings to other demographic and general populations. A notable limitation of our study is related to the temporal scope of the data utilized in our study. The dataset stems from the WHEL study conducted between 1995 and 2000, prompting concerns regarding its applicability to the current context in 2023. It's reasonable to acknowledge that the social landscape and lifestyle patterns have likely evolved over the past two decades. Despite this, we assert that certain fundamental physiological processes influenced by living alone and physical health remain the same. For instance, the well-established connection between physical health and mortality is less prone to drastic alterations over time. In addition, it's crucial to bring attention to the prevailing trend of increased prevalence in individuals living alone, as evidenced by refs. [6,10]. This noteworthy rise in solitary living defies assumptions and emphasizes the ongoing relevance and importance of our research topic. In this contemporary context, the physiological and health implications of living alone might hold even greater significance, given the heightened prevalence of this living arrangement. Regarding the temporal extent of data collection, it's worth noting that while the baseline data was collected between 1995 and 2000, the study encompassed a follow-up period extending until 2006, and the death index was updated until 2009. This extended data collection duration affords us a broader range of information over time, potentially offering insights into the dynamics and changes that occurred during this period.

We acknowledge that our findings may serve as preliminary data, laying the groundwork for future research endeavors. As such, we encourage future studies to build upon our work, ideally utilizing more recent and comprehensive datasets that encompass a broader spectrum of variables and an extended follow-up period. Given the current lack of consensus on the concept of social isolation in cancer populations, it is recommended that further research be conducted to consider the development and implementation of new social isolation assessment tools that encompass both subjective and objective measures of social isolation [26,27]. Furthermore, we suggest implementing community-based interventions that foster social connections and physical activity. These interventions may involve initiatives like revitalizing public spaces or establishing community exercise programs, as supported by previous studies [4,28–31].

5. Conclusions

This study highlights the significant joint impact of living alone and physical health on the mortality of breast cancer survivors, emphasizing the importance of addressing this social issue—living alone. Healthcare professionals should be aware of the living arrangements of cancer survivor patients, particularly if they are living alone. It is crucial for healthcare professionals, including nurses and physicians, to utilize social isolation assessment tools that are specifically designed for cancer survivors. This approach is vital in delivering precise and tailored care to meet the unique needs of these patients. Moreover, with a mindful acknowledgment of the unique health effects tied to living alone, healthcare administrators and policymakers can devise approaches fostering increased opportunities for community socialization and physical activity. This might entail enhancing access to green and public spaces, especially in urban marginalized communities prone to experiencing collective isolation, which could decrease the mortality risk from breast cancer [31–33].

Author Contributions: Conceptualization, T.W.; methodology, T.W. and C.D.; software, C.D., T.W. and F.-C.H.; validation, T.W., C.D., H.L. and F.-C.H.; formal analysis, C.D., T.W. and H.L.; resources, J.P.P. and T.W.; data curation, C.D. and T.W.; writing—original draft preparation, C.D.; writing—review and editing, C.D., T.W. and E.K.; visualization, C.D.; supervision, T.W.; project administration, T.W.; funding acquisition, T.W. All authors have read and agreed to the published version of the manuscript.

Funding: This research is partially supported by California Tobacco-Related Disease Research Program (TRDRP)—T30IP0998 and San Diego State University state funds. The WHEL study was initiated with the support of the Walton Family Foundation and continued with funding from the National Cancer Institute grant CA 69375. Cassandra Marie Doyle is supported by Wu's student award from TRDRP—Cornelius Hopper Diversity Award.

Institutional Review Board Statement: We use de-identified data; thus, the IRB review was exempt. The exempt IRB was approved by the San Diego State University IRB committee (protocol number: Temp-1286).

Informed Consent Statement: Inform consent was obtained from all subjects in the original WHEL cohort.

Data Availability Statement: Most of the data used in this paper can be found at: https://library.ucsd.edu/dc/object/bb2493244b (accessed on 18 April 2022).

Conflicts of Interest: The authors declare no conflict of interest.

References

1. Survivorship: During and after Treatment. Available online: https://www.cancer.org/cancer/survivorship.html (accessed on 18 August 2023).
2. Key Statistics for Breast Cancer. Available online: https://www.cancer.org/cancer/types/breast-cancer/about/how-common-is-breast-cancer.html (accessed on 18 August 2023).
3. Lee, I.; Park, C. The mediating effect of social support on uncertainty in illness and quality of life of female cancer survivors: A cross-sectional study. *Health Qual. Life Outcomes* **2020**, *18*, 143. [CrossRef]
4. Nicolaus, T. Building social connectedness vital for public health. *Nation's Health* **2023**, *53*, 1–14.
5. Hodgson, S.; Watts, I.; Fraser, S.; Roderick, P.; Dambha-Miller, H. Loneliness, social isolation, cardiovascular disease and mortality: A synthesis of the literature and conceptual framework. *J. R. Soc. Med.* **2020**, *113*, 185–192. [CrossRef]
6. Holt-Lunstad, J.; Smith, T.B.; Baker, M.; Harris, T.; Stephenson, D. Loneliness and social isolation as risk factors for mortality: A meta-analytic review. *Perspect. Psychol. Sci.* **2015**, *10*, 227–237. [CrossRef] [PubMed]
7. Paul, E.; Bu, F.; Fancourt, D. Loneliness and Risk for Cardiovascular Disease: Mechanisms and Future Directions. *Curr. Cardiol. Rep.* **2021**, *23*, 68. [CrossRef] [PubMed]
8. Brown, J.C.; Harhay, M.O.; Harhay, M.N. Physical function as a prognostic biomarker among cancer survivors. *Br. J. Cancer* **2015**, *112*, 194–198. [CrossRef]
9. Kroenke, C.H.; Kubzansky, L.D.; Schernhammer, E.S.; Holmes, M.D.; Kawachi, I. Social Networks, Social Support, and Survival After Breast Cancer Diagnosis. *J. Clin. Oncol.* **2006**, *24*, 1105–1111. [CrossRef]
10. Census Bureau Releases New Estimates on America's Families and Living Arrangements. 2021. Available online: https://www.census.gov/newsroom/press-releases/2021/families-and-living-arrangements.html (accessed on 18 April 2023).
11. Hinzey, A.; Gaudier-Diaz, M.M.; Lustberg, M.B.; Devries, A.C. Breast cancer and social environment: Getting by with a little help from our friends. *Breast Cancer Res.* **2016**, *18*, 54. [CrossRef]
12. Abell, J.G.; Steptoe, A. Living alone and mortality: More complicated than it seems. *Eur. Heart J. Qual. Care Clin. Outcomes* **2019**, *5*, 187–188. [CrossRef]
13. Elovainio, M.; Lumme, S.; Arffman, M.; Manderbacka, K.; Pukkala, E.; Hakulinen, C. Living alone as a risk factor for cancer incidence, case-fatality and all-cause mortality: A nationwide registry study. *SSM Popul. Health* **2021**, *15*, 100826. [CrossRef]
14. Kroenke, C.H.; Paskett, E.D.; Cené, C.W.; Caan, B.J.; Luo, J.; Shadyab, A.H.; Robinson, J.R.; Nassir, R.; Lane, D.S.; Anderson, G.L. Prediagnosis social support, social integration, living status, and colorectal cancer mortality in postmenopausal women from the women's health initiative. *Cancer* **2020**, *126*, 1766–1775. [CrossRef] [PubMed]
15. Nakano, J.; Fukushima, T.; Tanaka, T.; Fu, J.B.; Morishita, S. Physical function predicts mortality in patients with cancer: A systematic review and meta-analysis of observational studies. *Support. Care Cancer* **2021**, *29*, 5623–5634. [CrossRef]
16. Pierce, J.P.; Faerber, S.; Wright, F.A.; Rock, C.L.; Newman, V.; Flatt, S.W.; Kealey, S.; Jones, V.E.; Caan, B.J.; Gold, E.B.; et al. A randomized trial of the effect of a plant-based dietary pattern on additional breast cancer events and survival: The Women's Healthy Eating and Living (WHEL) Study. *Control Clin. Trials* **2002**, *23*, 728–756. [CrossRef]
17. Hays, R.D.; Morales, L.S. The RAND-36 measure of health-related quality of life. *Ann. Med.* **2001**, *33*, 350–357. [CrossRef] [PubMed]
18. Ware, J.E., Jr.; Sherbourne, C.D. The MOS 36-Item Short-Form Health Survey (SF-36): I. Conceptual Framework and Item Selection. *Med. Care* **1992**, *30*, 473–483. [CrossRef]
19. Item Short Form Survey (SF-36) Scoring Instructions. Available online: https://www.rand.org/health-care/surveys_tools/mos/36-item-short-form/scoring.html (accessed on 18 April 2023).
20. Tessou, K.D.; Lemus, H.; Hsu, F.-C.; Pierce, J.; Hong, S.; Brown, L.; Wu, T. Independent and Joint Impacts of Acid-Producing Diets and Depression on Physical Health among Breast Cancer Survivors. *Nutrients* **2021**, *13*, 2422. [CrossRef]
21. Pierce, J.P.; Natarajan, L.; Caan, B.J.; Parker, B.A.; Greenberg, E.R.; Flatt, S.W.; Rock, C.L.; Kealey, S.; Al-Delaimy, W.; Bardwell, W.A.; et al. Influence of a Diet Very High in Vegetables, Fruit, and Fiber and Low in Fat on Prognosis Following Treatment for Breast Cancer: The Women's Healthy Eating and Living (WHEL) randomized trial. *JAMA* **2007**, *298*, 289–298. [CrossRef] [PubMed]
22. Johnson-Kozlow, M.; Rock, C.L.; Gilpin, E.A.; Hollenbach, K.A.; Pierce, J.P. Validation of the WHI brief physical activity questionnaire among women diagnosed with breast cancer. *Am. J. Health Behav.* **2007**, *31*, 193–202. [CrossRef]
23. Hong, S.; Bardwell, W.A.; Natarajan, L.; Flatt, S.W.; Rock, C.L.; Newman, V.A.; Madlensky, L.; Mills, P.J.; Dimsdale, J.E.; Thomson, C.A.; et al. Correlates of physical activity level in breast cancer survivors participating in the Women's Healthy Eating and Living (WHEL) Study. *Breast Cancer Res. Treat.* **2007**, *101*, 225–232. [CrossRef]
24. Wei, M.Y.; Kabeto, M.U.; Galecki, A.T.; Langa, K.M. Physical Functioning Decline and Mortality in Older Adults With Multimorbidity: Joint Modeling of Longitudinal and Survival Data. *J. Gerontol. Ser. A* **2019**, *74*, 226–232. [CrossRef]

25. Saquib, N.; Pierce, J.P.; Saquib, J.; Flatt, S.W.; Natarajan, L.; Bardwell, W.A.; Patterson, R.E.; Stefanick, M.L.; Thomson, C.A.; Rock, C.L.; et al. Poor physical health predicts time to additional breast cancer events and mortality in breast cancer survivors. *Psycho-Oncology* **2011**, *20*, 252–259. [CrossRef]
26. Liang, Y.; Hao, G.; Wu, M.; Hou, L. Social isolation in adults with cancer: An evolutionary concept analysis. *Front. Psychol.* **2022**, *13*, 973640. [CrossRef] [PubMed]
27. National Academies of Sciences Engineering and Medicine (U.S.). Committee on the Health and Medical Dimensions of Social Isolation and Loneliness in Older Adults. In *Social Isolation and Loneliness in Older Adults: Opportunities for the Health Care System, in Consensus Study Report*; National Academies Press: Washington, DC, USA, 2020.
28. Knobf, M.T.; Thompson, A.S.; Fennie, K.; Erdos, D.M. The Effect of a Community-Based Exercise Intervention on Symptoms and Quality of Life. *Cancer Nurs.* **2014**, *37*, E43–E50. [CrossRef] [PubMed]
29. Leach, H.; Danyluk, J.; Culos–Reed, S. Design and Implementation of a Community-Based Exercise Program for Breast Cancer Patients. *Curr. Oncol.* **2014**, *21*, 267–271. [CrossRef] [PubMed]
30. Rief, W.; Bardwell, W.A.; Dimsdale, J.E.; Natarajan, L.; Flatt, S.W.; Pierce, J.P. Long-term course of pain in breast cancer survivors: A 4-year longitudinal study. *Breast Cancer Res. Treat.* **2011**, *130*, 579–586. [CrossRef] [PubMed]
31. Shirazipour, C.H.; Raines, C.; Liu, E.; Ruggieri, R.M.; Capaldi, J.M.; Luna-Lupercio, B.; Diniz, M.A.; Gresham, G.; Bhowmick, N.; Haile, R.W.; et al. Benefits of nature-based walking for breast cancer survivors. *BMJ Open* **2023**, *13*, e071041. [CrossRef]
32. Dawe, J.C. How Public Spaces Can Help Combat Urban Loneliness. 2021. Available online: https://www.salzburgglobal.org/news/latest-news/article/how-public-spaces-can-help-combat-urban-loneliness#:~:text=Access%20to%20green%20and%20public,social%20connection%20and%20support%20networks (accessed on 18 April 2023).
33. Rodriguez-Loureiro, L.; Verdoodt, F.; Lefebvre, W.; Vanpoucke, C.; Casas, L.; Gadeyne, S. Long-term exposure to residential green spaces and site-specific cancer mortality in urban Belgium: A 13-year follow-up cohort study. *Environ. Int.* **2022**, *170*, 107571. [CrossRef]

Disclaimer/Publisher's Note: The statements, opinions and data contained in all publications are solely those of the individual author(s) and contributor(s) and not of MDPI and/or the editor(s). MDPI and/or the editor(s) disclaim responsibility for any injury to people or property resulting from any ideas, methods, instructions or products referred to in the content.

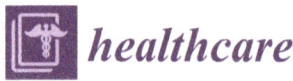

Article

Preferred Place of End-of-Life Care Based on Clinical Scenario: A Cross-Sectional Study of a General Japanese Population

Kyoko Hanari [1,2], Sandra Y. Moody [1,3,4], Takehiro Sugiyama [1,5,6,7,*] and Nanako Tamiya [1,5]

1. Health Services Research and Development Center, University of Tsukuba, Tsukuba City 305-8575, Japan
2. Hinohara Memorial Peace House Hospital, Nakai 259-0151, Japan
3. Department of Post-Graduate Education, Kameda Medical Center, Kamogawa City 296-0041, Japan
4. Department of Medicine, Division of Geriatrics, University of California, San Francisco, CA 94143, USA
5. Department of Health Services Research, Institute of Medicine, University of Tsukuba, Tsukuba 305-8575, Japan
6. Diabetes and Metabolism Information Center, Research Institute, National Center for Global Health and Medicine, Tokyo 162-8655, Japan
7. Institute for Global Health Policy Research, Bureau of International Health Cooperation, National Center for Global Health and Medicine, Tokyo 162-8655, Japan
* Correspondence: tsugiyama@md.tsukuba.ac.jp; Tel.: +81-29-853-8324

Abstract: In Japan, which has an aging society with many deaths, it is important that people discuss preferred place for end-of-life care in advance. This study aims to investigate whether the preferred place of end-of-life care differs by the assumed clinical scenario. This clinical scenario-based survey used data from a nationwide survey conducted in Japan in December 2017. Participants aged 20 years and older were randomly selected from the general population. The survey contained questions based on three scenarios: cancer, end-stage heart disease, and dementia. For each scenario, respondents were asked to choose the preferred place of end-of-life care among three options: home, nursing home, and medical facility. Eight hundred eighty-nine individuals participated in this study (effective response rate: 14.8%). The proportions of respondents choosing home, nursing home, and medical facility for the cancer scenario were 49.6%, 10.9%, and 39.5%, respectively; for the end-stage heart disease scenario, 30.5%, 18.9%, and 50.6%; and for the dementia scenario, 15.2%, 54.5%, and 30.3% ($p < 0.0001$, chi-square test). The preferred place of end-of-life care differed by the assumed clinical scenario. In clinical practice, concrete information about diseases and their status should be provided during discussions about preferred place for end-of-life care to reveal people's preferences more accurately.

Keywords: advance care planning; end of life; general population; preferred place of care; clinical scenario-based survey

Citation: Hanari, K.; Moody, S.Y.; Sugiyama, T.; Tamiya, N. Preferred Place of End-of-Life Care Based on Clinical Scenario: A Cross-Sectional Study of a General Japanese Population. *Healthcare* 2023, 11, 406. https://doi.org/10.3390/healthcare11030406

Academic Editor: Hidetaka Hamasaki

Received: 29 December 2022
Revised: 23 January 2023
Accepted: 27 January 2023
Published: 31 January 2023

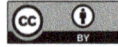

Copyright: © 2023 by the authors. Licensee MDPI, Basel, Switzerland. This article is an open access article distributed under the terms and conditions of the Creative Commons Attribution (CC BY) license (https://creativecommons.org/licenses/by/4.0/).

1. Introduction

The Japanese population is aging [1]; the Japanese Ministry of Health, Labour and Welfare (MHLW) is building a system that can comprehensively provide medical and nursing care in the community [2]. It is expected that the number of deaths in old age will further increase in the future [1]; however, a previous study showed the prevalence of incapacity to consent to treatment or admission was 45% for a psychiatric setting and 34% for a medical setting [3]. Healthcare providers may not be aware of a person's medical and nursing care preferences and, as a result, may provide unintended medical or nursing care. Therefore, it is essential to promote advance care planning (ACP). ACP is the process of understanding and sharing a person's preferences regarding future medical treatment and care [4,5]. Its goal is to coordinate preferences for care with the care received [6]. It is especially important for people to discuss, in advance, the place of care during the end of life, because it is believed that dying in a preferred place is an important aspect of a good death for both patients and their families [7]. Despite these advantages, even if some individuals with an illness can hold a discussion with other people, other individuals may not necessarily accept engaging in ACP due to barriers such as prognostic uncertainty, insufficient time during clinical encounters, poor knowledge about ACP, and physician communication skills [8–10]. Therefore, it is important to start ACP and think about the preferred place of end-of-life care before people become incapable of making decisions for themselves.

Several studies have shown that the home is the most frequently preferred place of end-of-life care (31–84%) among the general population [11–16]. These research results have had a stimulating effect on policies to promote home care. Although about half of people preferred home as a place of care, the rest preferred other places in general. The proportion of deaths at home in Japan was 15.7% in 2020 [17], and one of the reasons for this may be that some people do not want to receive medical or nursing care at home. Thus, it is important to clarify which factors are associated with choosing the preferred place of care. Previous studies have shown that the preferred place of care was associated with age [12,18], sex [11,18], marital status [13], concern about family burden [18], life experiences (education, hospitalization of a relative, perceived ability to get better pain relief, and longer hospitalization) [12], and familiarity with home care in the general population [11]. In these and other previous studies, respondents were not asked about their preferred place of end-of-life care in the context of a specific disease. Therefore, it remains unclear whether the preferred place of end-of-life care differs according to the assumed clinical scenario. We hypothesized that the preferred place of care would differ depending on the clinical scenario, due to the differences in symptoms that can generally occur depending on the disease. If the preferred place of end-of-life care varies by the assumed clinical scenario, it would be important to include concrete scenarios of a disease in discussions with people. If it becomes clear that the preferred place of care differs depending on the assumed disease, it may be necessary to formulate a policy to improve the system for providing medical and nursing care not only at home but also at places other than home. Accordingly, the purpose of this study is to investigate whether the preferred place of end-of-life care differs by the assumed clinical scenario.

2. Materials and Methods

2.1. Study Design and Participants

In this cross-sectional study, we used data from the Survey of Public Attitude toward Medical Care at the End of Life, a nationwide population-based survey conducted by the MHLW in December 2017. This survey was conducted by the MHLW every five years to investigate interest in and attitude toward the end of life in the general population. The survey was administered to a nationally representative sample of the general population in Japan aged 20 years and over. The survey used a stratified two-stage random sampling method. In the first stage, 150 sites were randomly selected from the 2015 census enumeration district so that the number of samples at each site was about 20 to 47. In the second stage, individuals who were mailed surveys were randomly selected from the basic resident registers of each of the 150 sites. The survey was mailed to 6000 individuals along with a return envelope and a letter from the MHLW explaining the study, followed by reminders to nonrespondents a maximum of two times.

All the survey data obtained from the MHLW were anonymized. Consent was assumed if the participant chose to complete the survey. The study protocol was approved by the Institutional Review Board of the University of Tsukuba (approval no. 1254, date 30 October 2017).

2.2. Measures

2.2.1. Dependent Variable

Our dependent variable was the preferred place of end-of-life care chosen from among home, nursing home, or medical facility. We used questions that contained disease scenarios to investigate whether the preferred place of end-of-life care differed by the assumed clinical scenario.

2.2.2. Main Predictors

The main predictors were the assumed clinical scenario in which the respondents were asked the following questions based on three disease scenarios. Scenario 1 (cancer) stated, "Where would be your preferred place to receive care if you had terminal cancer, could not eat well, felt short of breath but had no pain, and your consciousness is alert and [you were] able to make decisions?" Scenario 2 (end-stage heart disease) stated, "Where would be your preferred place to receive care if you had end-stage heart disease and needed support eating meals, changing your clothes, and toileting, but your consciousness was alert and [you were] able to make decisions?" Scenario 3 (dementia) stated, "Where would be your preferred place to receive care if you had terminal dementia and had difficulty knowing where you were and recognizing your family members, and needed support eating meals, changing clothes, and toileting?" The words "terminal" or "end-stage" were included in each question to mean that the condition was incurable, and that the prognosis was less than one year. For each scenario, respondents selected one of three options: home, nursing home (i.e., long-term care facility), or medical facility (i.e., hospital). In Japan, a nursing home is a facility that provides 24-h operational support and cares for persons who require assistance with activities of daily living and who often have complex health needs and increased vulnerability [19]. A medical facility includes hospitals that provide medical care, such as medical wards, surgical wards, intensive care units, palliative care units, and nursing wards intended for home discharge preparation.

2.2.3. Potential Associated Variables

Demographic characteristics (age, sex, living arrangements, and academic attainment), presence or absence of a family doctor, experience caring for a loved one, the experience of the death of a loved one, and discussion of future treatment were included as potentially associated variables. These variables were chosen because on previous studies [11,20,21]; preferred place of care was associated with age, marital status, education level, end-of-life preparations, and experiences related to death and dying. Age was categorized as decades, starting with ages 20–29 and ending with age 80 or over. The response categories for education level were "elementary school", "high school", "junior college", "bachelor's degree", and "graduate school". The survey did not ask respondents about their household income or other health conditions.

2.3. Statistical Analysis

Descriptive statistics examined baseline characteristics, including demographic characteristics (age, sex, living arrangements, and academic attainment), presence or absence of a family doctor, experience caring for a loved one, the experience of the death of a loved one, and discussion of future treatment.

Next, we illustrated the proportion of the preferred place of end-of-life care for each scenario. We examined whether the distribution of preferred place of end-of-life care was uniform using the chi-square test with four degrees of freedom. We then investigated the effect modification of the association between the assumed clinical scenario and the preferred place of end-of-life care by sex and age (<65 and $\geq$65 years), based on the definition by the Japan Geriatrics Society [22] and the Health Care Insurance System [23]). We tested effect modification using the likelihood-ratio test and the Wald test. For the likelihood-ratio test, we constructed (i) a multinomial logistic regression model to investigate the association of preferred place of care and hypothetical disease and sex or age and (ii) a multinomial logistic regression model with a product term of hypothetical disease and sex or age to address the effect modification, which was followed by the likelihood-ratio test between models (i) and (ii). We considered clustering answers by individuals using generalized estimating equations for the Wald test. Then, we performed the Wald test to examine the homogeneity of the proportional distribution by age or sex.

All statistics were performed using Stata® 15 (StataCorp, College Station, TX, USA). The level of statistical significance was set at $p < 0.05$.

3. Results

There were 973 respondents. Listwise deletion was used to exclude responses with missing values of age, sex, and preferred place of care. Data for 889 respondents, equivalent to 91.4%, were analyzed, giving an effective response rate of 14.8% on the national survey from which our data were drawn. Details of the selection process are shown in Figure 1.

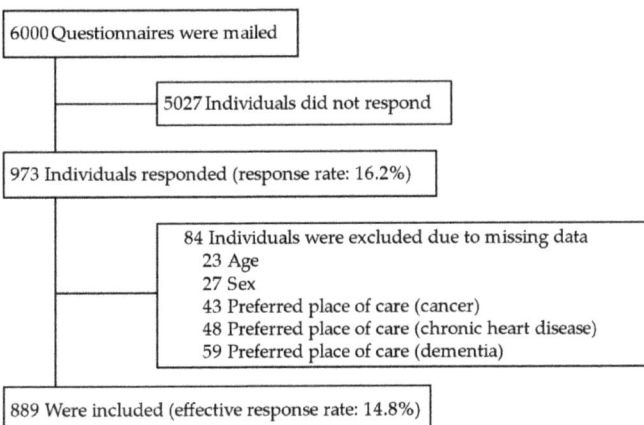

Figure 1. Flowchart of respondents. The 84 individuals missed at least one of the variables; the total number of missingness, therefore, exceeded 84.

Table 1 shows the characteristics of the respondents. Less than half (53.1%) were aged 60 and older, 56.0% were men, and most (81.8%) lived with at least one family member. Nearly 55% had at least a junior college education. Less than half had a primary physician (40.9%), 37.4% experienced caring for a loved one, 41.7% experienced the death of a loved one, and 39.5% discussed future treatment if they had a severe illness.

Table 1. Characteristics of the respondents, N = 889.

Characteristics	N (%)
Age, years	
<65	492 (55.3)
≥65	397 (44.7)
By decade	
20–29	39 (4.4)
30–39	107 (12.1)
40–49	137 (15.4)
50–59	133 (15.0)
60–69	188 (21.1)
70–79	188 (21.1)
≥80	97 (10.9)
Sex	
Men	498 (56.0)
Women	391 (44.0)
Education	
Elementary school	92 (10.4)
High school	306 (34.4)
Junior college	171 (19.2)
Bachelor's degree or graduate school	317 (35.7)
No answer	3 (0.3)

Table 1. Cont.

Characteristics	N (%)
Living arrangements	
Alone	142 (16.0)
With ≥1 family member	727 (81.8)
No answer	20 (2.2)
Has a family doctor	
Yes	364 (40.9)
No	518 (58.3)
No answer	7 (0.8)
Experience caring for a loved one	
Yes	332 (37.4)
No	549 (61.7)
No answer	8 (0.9)
Experienced death of a loved one	
Yes	371 (41.7)
No	484 (54.4)
No answer	34 (3.8)
Discussed future treatment	
Yes	351 (39.5)
No	505 (56.8)
No answer	33 (3.7)

The preferred place of care in the assumed clinical scenario is shown in Figure 2. Preferred place of end-of-life care differed by the clinical scenario, because the distributions were statistically significantly different for each clinical scenario ($p < 0.0001$, chi-square test). For the assumed clinical scenario of cancer, most (49.6%) respondents chose home as a preferred place to receive end-of-life care compared with a nursing home (10.9%) or a medical facility (39.5%). For end-stage heart disease, a medical facility was most often chosen (50.6%). For dementia, a nursing home was commonly chosen (54.5%). Additional analyzes also showed that the preferred places of care actually selected were deviated from expectations in each disease (Table S1).

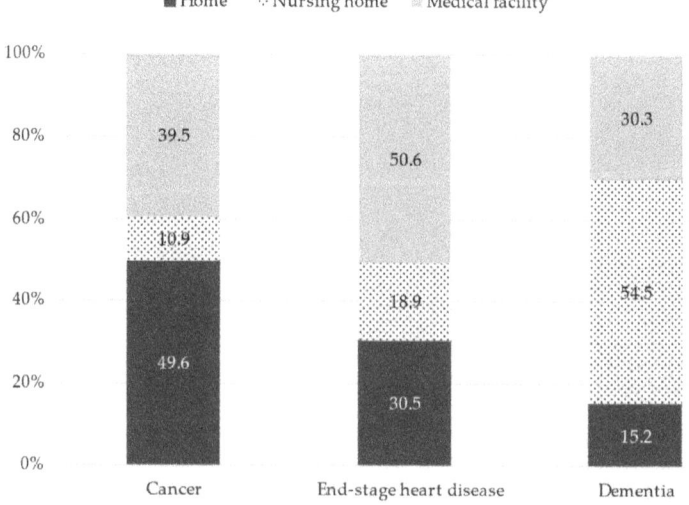

Figure 2. Proportion of preferred place of care by assumed clinical scenario, N = 889.

The preferred place of care by the assumed clinical scenario stratified by age or sex is shown in Figures 3 and 4, respectively. For age, the proportion who chose home in the assumed clinical scenario of cancer by age <65 and ≥65 was 53.8% vs. 44.3%, medical facility by the scenario of end-stage heart disease was 51.2% vs. 49.9%, and nursing home by the scenario of dementia was 64.8% vs. 41.8%. There was an effect modification by age (likelihood-ratio test, $p < 0.001$; Wald test, $p < 0.001$) but not by sex (likelihood-ratio test, $p = 0.21$; Wald test, $p = 0.06$) for the association between the assumed clinical scenario and the preferred place of end-of-life care. When the relationship between the preferred place of care and the assumed clinical scenario of dementia was examined by age, those <65 were significantly more likely to choose a nursing home and not home compared to a medical facility, but when end-stage heart disease was examined, those <65 were not likely to choose home compared to a medical facility.

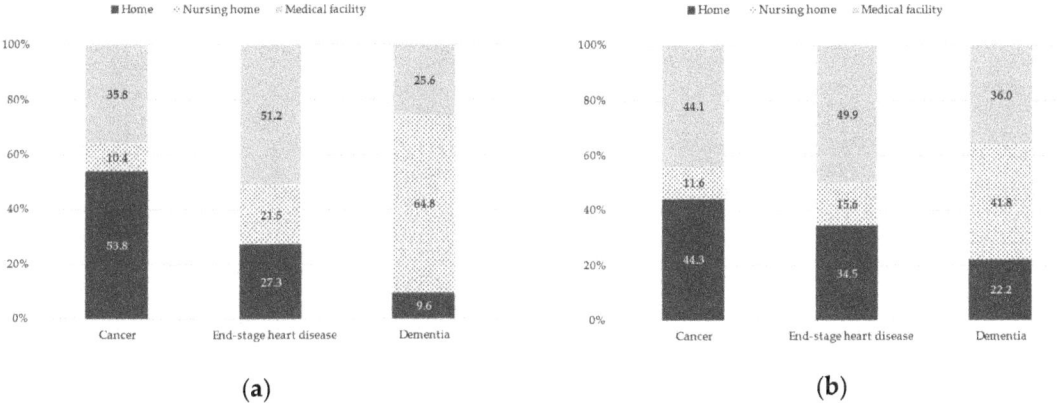

Figure 3. Proportion of preferred place of care by assumed clinical scenario stratified by age: (a) Age < 65 (n = 492); (b) Age ≥ 65 (n = 397). Likelihood-ratio test: $p < 0.001$, Wald test: $p < 0.001$.

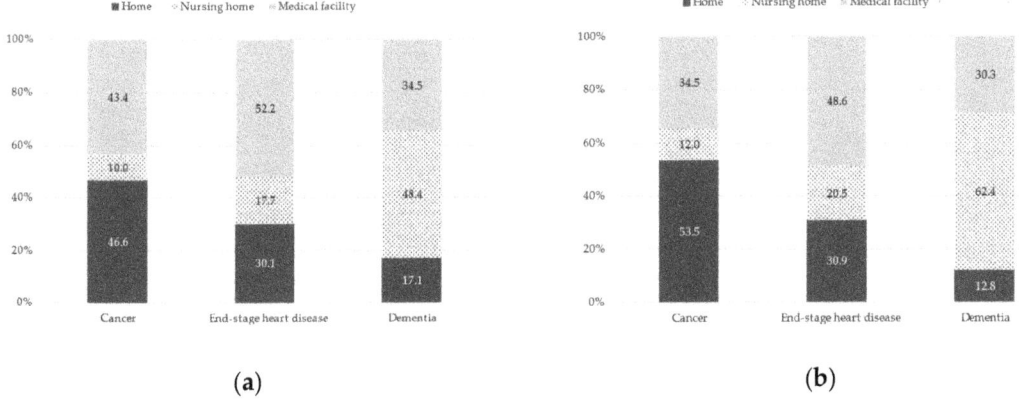

Figure 4. Proportion of preferred place of care by assumed clinical scenario stratified by sex: (a) Men (n = 498); (b) Women (n = 391). Likelihood-ratio test: $p = 0.21$, Wald test: $p = 0.06$.

4. Discussion

In this study, we investigated the differences between the preferred place of end-of-life care according to three assumed clinical scenarios among the general population in Japan. Respondents chose their preferred place of end-of-life care based on the three scenarios. For the assumed clinical scenario of cancer, the largest percentage of respondents chose their home as a preferred place to receive care at the end of life. However, medical facilities were most often chosen if respondents had end-stage heart disease, and nursing homes were chosen in the dementia scenario. As these distributions showed statistically significant differences, the results suggest preferred place of end-of-life care differs by the clinical scenario. In addition, our findings suggest that the relationship between the preferred place of care and the assumed clinical scenario is modified by age. Previous population-based studies that investigated preferred places of end-of-life care did not include the assumed clinical scenario as a variable. In this setting, a home was most often chosen as the preferred place of end-of-life care [11,14,15,18]. To our knowledge, this is the first study to show that the preferred place of end-of-life care differs by the assumed clinical scenario. The results suggest that providing concrete information about a disease during discussions about a preferred place of end-of-life care more accurately reveals people's preferences. In addition, these results are important because they may suggest that it is necessary to consider policies to promote the enrichment of end-of-life care, not only at home, but also at places other than home.

Potential explanations for the association between the assumed clinical scenario and the preferred place of end-of-life care include the following. First, we believe the difference in preferred place of care based on the assumed clinical scenario might be associated with knowledge about and images of each disease included in the scenario. For the assumed clinical scenario of cancer, the largest percentage of respondents chose home as a preferred place of end-of-life care, which is consistent with previous studies [18,24]. In Japan, when people think of end-stage cancer, they may imagine that end-of-life care is best provided in their homes, surrounded by family members. This is likely true, because previous studies that investigated components which might contribute to a good death in cancer care in Japan showed that spending enough time with one's family, having family at one's bedside, living in calm circumstances, and living in a home-like environment may contribute to a good death [20].

In contrast, when people think about end-stage heart disease, they assume that care should be provided in a medical facility because people believe that those with end-stage heart failure need intensive symptom management, including palliative care [25–27]. It is very likely that the general population might imagine that this care can only be provided in an inpatient setting. When dementia was considered, the largest percentage of respondents chose a nursing home as a preferred place of end-of-life care. The trajectory of dementia, in contrast to other diseases, is gradual and accompanied by a progressive decline in cognition and function [28,29]. When people think about end-stage dementia in Japan, they may believe that having end-stage dementia would be a burden on their family [30], and therefore would prefer nursing home placement to lessen the potential burden.

Other studies came to a different conclusion. Among those investigating the preferred place of care for patients [18,31,32], one study showed that patient preferences regarding place of care varied among their diagnoses [33]. As previous studies have shown, public opinion often does not coincide with the views of individuals who are close to death [34]. Moreover, the patient's health status may change over time, leading to changes in their preferences for care [35,36]. Accordingly, our findings have a few implications for clinical practice. When discussing the preferred place of end-of-life care in the future, including the assumed clinical scenario in the discussion may help a person better visualize their preference for the place of end-of-life care. It is certainly challenging to present all clinical scenarios when the preferred place of care is discussed with others. However, healthcare providers should consider raising the subject of common diseases that occur in the general population, such as dementia, cancer, and chronic heart or pulmonary disease, with different trajectories.

Second, we believe that the structure and funding of the healthcare system in Japan may influence people's preferences for the place of end-of-life care. In contrast to the United States, where hospice care is provided to all under the federal Medicare insurance program based on a life expectancy of fewer than six months irrespective of disease, in Japan, only patients with cancer or HIV diagnoses can be admitted to a palliative care unit. The United Kingdom, Germany, and Canada have similar systems to that of the United States. In addition, in Japan, when people are 65 and older, home care is provided under the Long-term Care Insurance (LTCI) system regardless of disease status; however, for those aged 40–64 years who need home care, the LTCI system will only cover 16 diseases (end-stage cancer and dementia are included). Knowledge of the LTCI system may influence people's choices of preferred places for end-of-life care. Therefore, healthcare providers in Japan should be aware of the possibility that patient knowledge about the healthcare system may have an impact on their choices for the preferred place of care. In addition, in countries where palliative care is available to all regardless of disease status, healthcare providers should be aware that the preferred place of care may differ based on the type of disease.

Last, our findings showed that the relationship between the preferred place of end-of-life care and the assumed clinical scenario is modified by age. When the relationship between the preferred place of care and the assumed clinical scenario of dementia was examined by age, those <65 were significantly more likely to choose a nursing home, and not home, compared to a medical facility, but when end-stage heart disease was examined, those <65 were not likely to choose home compared to a medical facility. Previous studies from Japan [11,12,18] indicated that those who were less than 65 years of age chose home as a place of end-of-life care compared to a medical facility; however, in those studies, the place was not selected after assuming the disease. The preferred place of care in the context of the assumed clinical scenario can change with age, and thus, it would be important to discuss the preferred place of end-of-life care repeatedly over time.

Our results did not show a significant difference in the preferred place of end-of-life care and the assumed clinical scenario based on sex, which was found in previous studies [11,18]. Interestingly, in the Wald test, which clustered answers by respondents, we found a smaller p-value with this test than in the likelihood-ratio test (no clustering), which indicates that each respondent's answers for the different scenarios were "dispersed" across the diseases, i.e., "different" rather than concentrated on one choice.

Limitations and Strengths

This study has several limitations. First, the study had a low response rate and was conducted in one country, making it difficult to generalize the results. In addition, we cannot rule out the possibility that the proportion of the preferred place of end-of-life care for each scenario would change due to selection bias, with those who are not interested in end-of-life care probably not responding to the survey. Although studies with high response rates are needed, low response rates and selection bias, as shown in Figure 2, do not seem to invalidate the results of this study. A second limitation is that the present study sampled the general population rather than patients with specific diseases; thus, our results may not be generalizable to a patient population. It is important to ask about preference for a place of end-of-life care to support the hopes of a person; however, the preferred place of end-of-life care does not necessarily correspond to better care, because each place has its limitations in terms of medical treatment provided or care received. Additionally, a previous study indicated that differences exist between pragmatic and ideal end-of-life preferences [35]. In actual discussions of the preferred place of end-of-life care with patients, healthcare providers need to consider the best place based on the patient's preferences as well as the status of the disease, symptomatology, and family situation. Third, we are unable to reveal whether the respondents chose the place of care according to the physical conditions or the specific disease in each clinical scenario. Additionally, we were unable to ascertain the reasons respondents chose a specific place of end-of-life care because questions addressing this issue were not included. Therefore, there is a need for surveys that include options that standardize physical conditions and differ only in naming the disease and studies that provide detailed reasons why respondents choose different places of end-of-life care. Finally, our study did not investigate effect modifications beyond age and sex. Previous studies have shown that marital status [13], concern about family burden [18], life experiences (education, hospitalization of a relative, perceived ability to get better pain relief, longer hospitalization) [12], and familiarity with home care [11] may influence people's choices of the preferred place of end-of-life care. Further studies evaluating these possible relationships may help us improve how the preferred place of end-of-life care is discussed with the general population.

The major strength of our study is that the same respondents selected each preferred place of end-of-life care while considering the assumed clinical scenario, which allowed us to examine how the assumed clinical scenario might influence people's choices. When the preferred place of care is discussed, providing concrete information about the disease or disease status would help people decide or better think about where they are at the end of life. Awareness of our findings on the part of policymakers could lead to policies that promote enhanced end-of-life care, not only at home but also at places other than at home.

5. Conclusions

The preferred place of end-of-life care differs by the assumed clinical scenario. More studies are needed to further elucidate the reasons for these choices. In clinical practice, providing concrete information about a patient's disease during discussions about a preferred place of end-of-life care is recommended for more accurately revealing a person's preferences. Additionally, regular discussions about a preferred place of end-of-life care may be important due to an effect modification by age for the association between the assumed clinical scenario and the preferred place of care. When formulating policies regarding the preferred place of end-of-life care among the general population, it is necessary to proceed with discussions based on an understanding that not only those who choose to remain in their own homes but also their preferred place may change depending on the assumed clinical scenario. Awareness of the findings here on the part of policymakers can lead to policies that promote enhanced end-of-life care, not only at home but also other than at home.

Supplementary Materials: The following supporting information can be downloaded at: https://www.mdpi.com/article/10.3390/healthcare11030406/s1. Table S1: The results of the chi-square test and Pearson's residual.

Author Contributions: K.H. and N.T. contributed to the study concept and design. Two authors (K.H. and N.T.) proposed several questions related to ACP to the MHLW that were included in the final survey. K.H. and N.T. contributed to the acquisition of data. K.H., S.Y.M., T.S. and N.T. contributed to the analysis and interpretation of the data. K.H. drafted the manuscript, and other authors critically reviewed and revised it for important intellectual content. All authors have read and agreed to the published version of the manuscript.

Funding: This research was funded by a grant-in-aid from the Ministry of Health, Labour and Welfare; Health and Labour Sciences Research Grant, Japan and Research on Regional Medicine (H28-iryou-ippan-013), and a grant-in-aid from the Ministry of Health, Labour and Welfare Policy Research Grants, Japan; Special Research (22CA2028). The sponsor did not contribute to the study design; the collection, analysis, and interpretation of data; the writing of the report; or the decision to submit the article for publication.

Institutional Review Board Statement: The study was conducted according to the guidelines of the Declaration of Helsinki and approved by the Institutional Review Board of the University of Tsukuba (approval no. 1254, date 30 October 2017).

Informed Consent Statement: Not applicable.

Data Availability Statement: The datasets used and analyzed during the current study are available from the corresponding author upon reasonable request.

Acknowledgments: The authors thank all participants who responded to this survey.

Conflicts of Interest: None of the authors of this manuscript have any conflict of interest (financial, personal, or potential conflict) to report.

References

1. Annual Health, Labour and Welfare Report 2021. Available online: https://www.mhlw.go.jp/english/wp/wp-hw14/index.html (accessed on 15 January 2023).
2. Iwagami, M.; Tamiya, N. The long-term care insurance system in Japan: Past, present, and future. *JMA J.* **2019**, *2*, 67–69. [CrossRef] [PubMed]
3. Lepping, P.; Stanly, T.; Turner, J. Systematic review on the prevalence of lack of capacity in medical and psychiatric settings. *Clin. Med.* **2015**, *15*, 337–343. [CrossRef]
4. Miyashita, J.; Shimizu, S.; Shiraishi, R.; Mori, M.; Okawa, K.; Aita, K.; Mitsuoka, S.; Nishikawa, K.; Kizawa, Y.; Morita, T.; et al. Culturally adapted consensus definition and action guideline: Japan's advance care planning. *J. Pain Symptom Manag.* **2022**, *64*, 602–613. [CrossRef] [PubMed]
5. Sudore, R.L.; Lum, H.D.; You, J.J.; Hanson, L.C.; Meier, D.E.; Pantilat, S.Z.; Matlock, D.D.; Rietjens, J.A.C.; Korfage, I.J.; Ritchie, C.S.; et al. Defining advance care planning for adults: A consensus definition from a multidisciplinary Delphi panel. *J. Pain Symptom Manag.* **2017**, *53*, 821–832.e1. [CrossRef] [PubMed]
6. Jimenez, G.; Tan, W.S.; Virk, A.K.; Low, C.K.; Car, J.; Ho, A.H.Y. Overview of systematic reviews of advance care planning: Summary of evidence and global lessons. *J. Pain Symptom Manag.* **2018**, *56*, 436–459.e25. [CrossRef] [PubMed]
7. Ikari, T.; Hiratsuka, Y.; Cheng, S.Y.; Miyashita, M.; Morita, T.; Mori, M.; Uneno, Y.; Amano, K.; Uehara, Y.; Yamaguchi, T.; et al. Factors associated with good death of patients with advanced cancer: A prospective study in Japan. *Support. Care Cancer* **2022**, *30*, 9577–9586. [CrossRef]
8. Peck, V.; Valiani, S.; Tanuseputro, P.; Mulpuru, S.; Kyeremanteng, K.; Fitzgibbon, E.; Forster, A.; Kobewka, D. Advance care planning after hospital discharge: Qualitative analysis of facilitators and barriers from patient interviews. *BMC Palliat. Care* **2018**, *17*, 127. [CrossRef]
9. Piers, R.D.; van Eechoud, I.J.; Van Camp, S.; Grypdonck, M.; Deveugele, M.; Verbeke, N.C.; Van Den Noortgate, N.J. Advance Care Planning in terminally ill and frail older persons. *Patient Educ. Couns.* **2013**, *90*, 323–329. [CrossRef]
10. Rosa, W.E.; Izumi, S.; Sullivan, D.R.; Lakin, J.; Rosenberg, A.R.; Creutzfeldt, C.J.; Lafond, D.; Tjia, J.; Cotter, V.; Wallace, C.; et al. Advance care planning in serious illness: A narrative review. *J. Pain Symptom Manag.* **2023**, *65*, e63–e78. [CrossRef]
11. Fukui, S.; Yoshiuchi, K.; Fujita, J.; Sawai, M.; Watanabe, M. Japanese people's preference for place of end-of-life care and death: A population-based nationwide survey. *J. Pain Symptom Manag.* **2011**, *42*, 882–892. [CrossRef]
12. Nishie, H.; Mizobuchi, S.; Suzuki, E.; Sato, K.; Toda, Y.; Matsuoka, J.; Morimatsu, H. Living will interest and preferred end-of-life care and death locations among Japanese adults 50 and over: A population-based survey. *Acta Med. Okayama* **2014**, *68*, 339–348. [CrossRef] [PubMed]
13. Wilson, D.M.; Cohen, J.; Deliens, L.; Hewitt, J.A.; Houttekier, D. The preferred place of last days: Results of a representative population-based public survey. *J. Palliat. Med.* **2013**, *16*, 502–508. [CrossRef] [PubMed]
14. Gomes, B.; Calanzani, N.; Gysels, M.; Hall, S.; Higginson, I.J. Heterogeneity and changes in preferences for dying at home: A systematic review. *BMC Palliat. Care* **2013**, *12*, 7. [CrossRef] [PubMed]
15. Chung, R.Y.; Wong, E.L.; Kiang, N.; Chau, P.Y.; Lau, J.Y.C.; Wong, S.Y.; Yeoh, E.K.; Woo, J.W. Knowledge, attitudes, and preferences of advance decisions, end-of-life care, and place of care and death in Hong Kong. A population-based telephone survey of 1067 adults. *J. Am. Med. Dir. Assoc.* **2017**, *18*, 367.e19–367.e27. [CrossRef]
16. Jiraphan, A.; Pitanupong, J. General population-based study on preferences towards end-of-life care in Southern Thailand: A cross-sectional survey. *BMC Palliat. Care* **2022**, *21*, 36. [CrossRef]
17. Ministry of Health, Labour and Welfare Number of Deaths, the Proportion of Place of Death. Available online: https://view.officeapps.live.com/op/view.aspx?src=https%3A%2F%2Fwww.mhlw.go.jp%2Ftoukei%2Fyouran%2Fdatar03k%2F1-25.xlsx&wdOrigin=BROWSELINK (accessed on 15 January 2023).
18. Yamagishi, A.; Morita, T.; Miyashita, M.; Yoshida, S.; Akizuki, N.; Shirahige, Y.; Akiyama, M.; Eguchi, K. Preferred place of care and place of death of the general public and cancer patients in Japan. *Support. Care Cancer* **2012**, *20*, 2575–2582. [CrossRef]
19. Sanford, A.M.; Orrell, M.; Tolson, D.; Abbatecola, A.M.; Arai, H.; Bauer, J.M.; Cruz-Jentoft, A.J.; Dong, B.; Ga, H.; Goel, A.; et al. An international definition for "nursing home". *J. Am. Med. Dir. Assoc.* **2015**, *16*, 181–184. [CrossRef]
20. Miyashita, M.; Sanjo, M.; Morita, T.; Hirai, K.; Uchitomi, Y. Good death in cancer care: A nationwide quantitative study. *Ann. Oncol.* **2007**, *18*, 1090–1097. [CrossRef]
21. Martin, R.S.; Hayes, B.; Gregorevic, K.; Lim, W.K. The effects of advance care planning interventions on nursing home residents: A systematic review. *J. Am. Med. Dir. Assoc.* **2016**, *17*, 284–293. [CrossRef]
22. Ouchi, Y.; Rakugi, H.; Arai, H.; Akishita, M.; Ito, H.; Toba, K.; Kai, I. Joint Committee of Japan Gerontological Society (JGLS) and Japan Geriatrics Society (JGS) on the definition and classification of the elderly Redefining the elderly as aged 75 years and older: Proposal from the Joint Committee of Japan Gerontological Society and the Japan Geriatrics Society. *Geriatr. Gerontol. Int.* **2017**, *17*, 1045–1047. [CrossRef]
23. Ministry of Health, Labour and Welfare Health Care Insurance System. Available online: https://www.mhlw.go.jp/english/wp/wp-hw5/dl/23010201e.pdf (accessed on 10 December 2022).
24. Sanjo, M.; Miyashita, M.; Morita, T.; Hirai, K.; Kawa, M.; Akechi, T.; Uchitomi, Y. Preferences regarding end-of-life cancer care and associations with good-death concepts: A population-based survey in Japan. *Ann. Oncol.* **2007**, *18*, 1539–1547. [CrossRef] [PubMed]

25. Yancy, C.W.; Jessup, M.; Bozkurt, B.; Butler, J.; Casey, D.E., Jr.; Colvin, M.M.; Drazner, M.H.; Filippatos, G.S.; Fonarow, G.C.; Givertz, M.M.; et al. 2017 ACC/AHA/HFSA Focused Update of the 2013 ACCF/AHA guideline for the management of heart failure: A report of the American College of Cardiology/American Heart Association Task Force on Clinical Practice guidelines and the Heart Failure Society of America. *Circulation* **2017**, *136*, e137–e161. [CrossRef] [PubMed]
26. Okumura, T.; Sawamura, A.; Murohara, T. Palliative and end-of-life care for heart failure patients in an aging society. *Korean J. Intern. Med.* **2018**, *33*, 1039–1049. [CrossRef] [PubMed]
27. McIlvennan, C.K.; Allen, L.A. Palliative care in patients with heart failure. *BMJ* **2016**, *353*, i1010. [CrossRef] [PubMed]
28. Sachs, G.A.; Shega, J.W.; Cox-Hayley, D. Barriers to excellent end-of-life care for patients with dementia. *J. Gen. Intern. Med.* **2004**, *19*, 1057–1063. [CrossRef]
29. Regier, N.G.; Hodgson, N.A.; Gitlin, L.N. Characteristics of activities for persons with dementia at the mild, moderate, and severe stages. *Gerontologist* **2017**, *57*, 987–997. [CrossRef]
30. Arai, Y.; Arai, A.; Zarit, S.H. What do we know about dementia?: A survey on knowledge about dementia in the general public of Japan. *Int. J. Geriatr. Psychiatry* **2008**, *23*, 433–438. [CrossRef]
31. Natsume, M.; Watanabe, K.; Matsumoto, S.; Naruge, D.; Hayashi, K.; Furuse, J.; Kawamura, M.; Jinno, H.; Sano, K.; Fukushima, R.; et al. Factors influencing cancer patients' choice of end-of-life care place. *J. Palliat. Med.* **2018**, *21*, 751–765. [CrossRef]
32. Wiggins, N.; Droney, J.; Mohammed, K.; Riley, J.; Sleeman, K.E. Understanding the factors associated with patients with dementia achieving their preferred place of death: A retrospective cohort study. *Age Ageing* **2019**, *48*, 433–439. [CrossRef]
33. Skorstengaard, M.H.; Neergaard, M.A.; Andreassen, P.; Brogaard, T.; Bendstrup, E.; Løkke, A.; Aagaard, S.; Wiggers, H.; Bech, P.; Jensen, A.B. Preferred place of care and death in terminally ill patients with lung and heart disease compared to cancer patients. *J. Palliat. Med.* **2017**, *20*, 1217–1224. [CrossRef]
34. Hoare, S.; Morris, Z.S.; Kelly, M.P.; Kuhn, I.; Barclay, S. Do patients want to die at home? A systematic review of the UK literature, focused on missing preferences for place of death. *PLoS ONE* **2015**, *10*, e0142723. [CrossRef] [PubMed]
35. Neergaard, M.A.; Brogaard, T.; Vedsted, P.; Jensen, A.B. Asking terminally ill patients about their preferences concerning place of care and death. *Int. J. Palliat. Nurs.* **2018**, *24*, 124–131. [CrossRef] [PubMed]
36. Evans, R.; Finucane, A.; Vanhegan, L.; Arnold, E.; Oxenham, D. Do place-of-death preferences for patients receiving specialist palliative care change over time? *Int. J. Palliat. Nurs.* **2014**, *20*, 579–583. [CrossRef] [PubMed]

Disclaimer/Publisher's Note: The statements, opinions and data contained in all publications are solely those of the individual author(s) and contributor(s) and not of MDPI and/or the editor(s). MDPI and/or the editor(s) disclaim responsibility for any injury to people or property resulting from any ideas, methods, instructions or products referred to in the content.

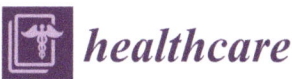

Article

Utilization of Primary Healthcare Services in Patients with Multimorbidity According to Their Risk Level by Adjusted Morbidity Groups: A Cross-Sectional Study in Chamartín District (Madrid)

Jaime Barrio-Cortes [1,2], Almudena Castaño-Reguillo [3], Beatriz Benito-Sánchez [1,*], María Teresa Beca-Martínez [2] and Cayetana Ruiz-Zaldibar [2]

1. Foundation for Biosanitary Research and Innovation in Primary Care (FIIBAP), 28003 Madrid, Spain
2. Faculty of Health, Camilo José Cela University, 28692 Madrid, Spain
3. Ciudad Jardín Health Center, Primary Care Management, 28002 Madrid, Spain
* Correspondence: beatrizbenitosanch@salud.madrid.org

Citation: Barrio-Cortes, J.; Castaño-Reguillo, A.; Benito-Sánchez, B.; Beca-Martínez, M.T.; Ruiz-Zaldibar, C. Utilization of Primary Healthcare Services in Patients with Multimorbidity According to Their Risk Level by Adjusted Morbidity Groups: A Cross-Sectional Study in Chamartín District (Madrid). *Healthcare* **2024**, *12*, 270. https://doi.org/10.3390/healthcare12020270

Academic Editors: Hidetaka Hamasaki and Aleksander Owczarek

Received: 17 November 2023
Revised: 16 January 2024
Accepted: 18 January 2024
Published: 20 January 2024

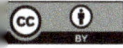

Copyright: © 2024 by the authors. Licensee MDPI, Basel, Switzerland. This article is an open access article distributed under the terms and conditions of the Creative Commons Attribution (CC BY) license (https://creativecommons.org/licenses/by/4.0/).

Abstract: Patients with multimorbidity have increased and more complex healthcare needs, posing their management a challenge for healthcare systems. This study aimed to describe their primary healthcare utilization and associated factors. A population-based cross-sectional study was conducted in a Spanish basic healthcare area including all patients with chronic conditions, differentiating between having multimorbidity or not. Sociodemographic, functional, clinical and service utilization variables were analyzed, stratifying the multimorbid population by the Adjusted Morbidity Groups (AMG) risk level, sex and age. A total of 6036 patients had multimorbidity, 64.2% being low risk, 28.5% medium risk and 7.3% high risk. Their mean age was 64.1 years and 63.5% were women, having on average 3.5 chronic diseases, and 25.3% were polymedicated. Their mean primary care contacts/year was 14.9 (7.8 with family doctors and 4.4 with nurses). Factors associated with primary care utilization were age (B-coefficient [BC] = 1.15; 95% Confidence Interval [CI] = 0.30–2.01), female sex (BC = 1.04; CI = 0.30–1.78), having a caregiver (BC = 8.70; CI = 6.72–10.69), complexity (B-coefficient = 0.46; CI = 0.38–0.55), high-risk (B-coefficient = 2.29; CI = 1.26–3.32), numerous chronic diseases (B-coefficient = 1.20; CI = 0.37–2.04) and polypharmacy (B-coefficient = 5.05; CI = 4.00–6.10). This study provides valuable data on the application of AMG in multimorbid patients, revealing their healthcare utilization and the need for a patient-centered approach by primary care professionals. These results could guide in improving coordination among professionals, optimizing multimorbidity management and reducing costs derived from their extensive healthcare utilization.

Keywords: multimorbidity; primary care; healthcare services utilization; patient management; morbidity grouper; stratification

1. Introduction

Multimorbidity is commonly defined as the presence of two or more chronic conditions in an individual [1–3]. There is no homogeneous universal definition for multimorbidity since it depends on the number, type and duration of the chronic diseases considered, as well as on the population and area studied and the data sources and data collection methods, among other factors [4].

The prevalence of chronic diseases has rapidly risen in the past years and is expected to continue increasing, and thus multimorbidity too. The main reasons are population aging and improvement in survival [5]. However, multimorbidity involves progressive clinical deterioration, increased disability, decline in quality and life expectancy, polypharmacy and increased health service utilization [1,2], especially in primary care [3].

Nowadays, multimorbidity poses a challenge for the management of patients with multimorbidity, as healthcare services usually focus on a single disease [3], leading to care that is sometimes inadequate and potentially harmful [1]. Therefore, patients with multimorbidity require novel multiple disease-specific strategies involving comprehensive and multidisciplinary patient-centered care, with disease-specific goals, together with careful prescription of multiple medications [1–3]. For designing a meaningful patient-centered approach, it is indispensable to characterize and understand the sequence of diseases, functional limitations and health service utilization of the population with multimorbidity, especially focusing on high-risk patients, in order to guide effective action for the improvement of clinical care and policy of patients with multimorbidity [6]. Nevertheless, there is still limited evidence to support any approach, so more research on multimorbidity is urgently needed [1].

The WHO has highlighted the fundamental role of primary care in the management of patients with multimorbidity [3,7]. To guide this management, many countries use morbidity groupers to stratify populations according to complexity [8]. In Spain, the Adjusted Morbidity Groups (AMGs) have been developed within the Spanish healthcare system and are integrated into the electronic medical records of primary care [9]. The AMG grouper enables the measurement of multimorbidity to determine its impact on clinical-care management, epidemiology and healthcare administration, while also classifying patients into risk categories based on their morbidity and complexity [10]. This tool is useful for primary care professionals and policymakers, as it reveals the characteristics and use of services in patients with multimorbidity, serving as a guide to allocate healthcare resources efficiently and to plan appropriate care models and interventions based on each individual risk level, thereby successfully meeting the healthcare needs of patients with multimorbidity and efficiently managing healthcare services [8–10].

As AMG is a relatively recent and useful tool, and as more research is needed to better characterize populations with multimorbidity for designing optimized care strategies, we aimed to describe the chronic conditions and the use of primary care services and associated factors in patients with multimorbidity according to their AMG risk level, sex and age, and comparing to those patients without multimorbidity.

2. Materials and Methods

2.1. Design, Setting and Study Subjects

A cross-sectional observational study was performed in a basic healthcare area located in the Chamartín district in Madrid (Spain). Chamartín is located in the north of Madrid city center and has 143,424 inhabitants, with an average age of 45 years (23% over 65 years), 55% women, 8.9% foreigners and corresponding to the lowest degree of socioeconomic deprivation. Madrid's healthcare system follows the Spanish National Health System, which guarantees almost universal coverage for all residents, organizing the healthcare management of the population by dividing the country into basic healthcare areas staffed by primary care teams under the gatekeeping model [11].

All the patients with chronic conditions were included in the study, differentiating between those without and with multimorbidity. The healthcare area studied covered 18,107 people, of whom 9886 had chronic illnesses as of 30 June 2015.

2.2. Data Collection

Data were requested from the Information Health Systems Department of Madrid Primary Care, which extracted all the study information registered in the Madrid primary care electronic medical record database for each chronic patient. Chronic patients were identified via the AMG tool in the electronic clinical record of the Madrid primary care system, which considers as chronic patients those who present at least one chronic disease listed in Table S1 [7].

2.3. Variables

AMG classifies populations considering morbidity and complexity. The AMG algorithm assigns a relative weight to mortality risk, admissions, primary care visits and prescriptions for the diagnostic code grouping present in each patient, allowing the calculation of an individual level of complexity depending on morbidity. The complexity numerical index obtained enables the stratification of the population into four risk levels following the Kaiser-Permanente pyramid, which assigns cut-off points from the 50th, 80th and 95th percentiles of the population, 50% of which corresponds to the to the population of people without any relevant chronic pathology, 30% to patients with chronic diseases and with low risk levels, 15% to those with medium risk, and 5% to those with high risk [9,10].

Sociodemographic variables including age, sex and country of origin (Spain, Europe or the rest of the world) were determined. Also, functional status was characterized by the presence of immobilization at home, institutionalization in a nursing home, requiring a primary caregiver, having home support and being in palliative care. Clinical characteristics were identified by AMG risk level (into low, medium or high risk), AMG complexity index (numerical value of patient complexity assigned by AMG), number and type of chronic diseases, multimorbidity (defined as suffering from at least two chronic conditions) and polymedication (defined the prescription of at least five medications for their chronic conditions). Regarding, primary care services utilization, the total number of annual contacts was calculated, as well as the number of contacts according to type (health, administrative, laboratory), form of contact (face-to-face, telephone, home visit) and professional contact (family physician, nurse, social worker, midwife, physiotherapist and dentist).

Sociodemographic, functional and clinical variables were extracted from Madrid's primary care electronic medical record database on 30 June 2015, while primary care service utilization was recorded from 30 June 2015 to 30 June 2016.

2.4. Statistical Analysis

To characterize the sample, descriptive statistics were calculated for all the variables in the study for the entire population with chronic diseases, as well as distinguishing between those suffering or not from multimorbidity, including the stratification of the multimorbid population by AMG risk level, sex and age group. Qualitative variables were described by counts and percentages, whereas quantitative variables were by means (standard deviation) or medians (interquartile range). Normality was measured with the Shapiro–Wilk test. For bivariate analysis, qualitative variables were compared via χ^2 tests (or Fisher's exact test when appropriate), and polytomous and quantitative variables with parametric or nonparametric tests. Multiple comparisons were adjusted by applying the Bonferroni correction. Factors associated with primary care utilization in the population with multimorbidity were identified by a multiple linear regression whose dependent variable was the total number of contacts with primary care and the independent variables those significantly associated with the total number of contacts with primary care determined in simple linear regression analyses. Results in bivariate and multivariable analyses were considered statistically significant if $p < 0.05$. Statistical analysis was performed with IBM SPSS Statistics version 25 software (IBM Corp., Armonk, NY, USA).

3. Results

In the healthcare area studied, 9866 (54.6%) patients had at least one chronic disease, and 6036 (33.3%) had multimorbidity. Patients with multimorbidity had a mean age of 64.1 years and 63.5% were women, while patients with only one chronic condition mean age was 42.6 and 58.1% were women. Regarding their functional status, 4.8% of patients with multimorbidity were immobilized, 2.4% institutionalized in a residence, 3.6% had a primary caregiver at home, 1.3% needed home support, and 0.7% received palliative care, these functional limitations being less frequent in patients with just one chronic disease. The mean number of chronic conditions in patients with multimorbidity was 3.5, and a total of 25.3% were polymedicated vs. 1.8% in chronic patients without multimorbidity and 64.2% were classified by AMG as low risk, 28.5% as medium risk and 7.3% as high-risk, whereas most chronic patients without multimorbidity were low-risk (Table 1).

Table 1. Sociodemographic, functional and clinical characteristics of the total population with chronic conditions and with or without multimorbidity.

Chronic Patients	Total	No Multimorbidity		Multimorbidity		p-Value
n (%)	9866 (100)	3830 (38.8)	95% CI	6036 (61.2)	95% CI	
Sociodemographic variables						
Female	6056 (61.4)	2225 (58.1)	56.5–59.6	3831 (63.5)	62.2–64.7	<0.001
Age *	55.7 (20.8)	42.6 (18.5)	42.1–43.2	64.1 (17.6)	63.6–64.5	<0.001
≤65 years	6383 (64.7)	3408 (89.0)	88.0–90.0	2975 (49.3)	48.0–50.5	<0.001
>65 years	3483 (35.3)	422 (11.0)	10.0–12.0	3061 (50.7)	49.4–51.9	
Origin Spain	8078 (81.9)	3026 (79.0)	77.7–80.3	5052 (83.7)	82.8–84.6	
Europe	367 (3.7)	178 (4.6)	3.9–5.3	189 (3.1)	2.7–3.6	<0.001
Rest of the world	1421 (14.4)	626 (16.3)	15.2–17.5	795 (13.2)	12.3–14.9	
Functional variables						
Immobilized	300 (3.0)	12 (0.3)	0.1–0.5	288 (4.8)	4.2–5.3	<0.001
Institutionalized	161 (1.6)	16 (0.4)	0.2–0.6	145 (2.4)	2.0–2.8	<0.001
Primary caregiver	229 (2.3)	9 (0.2)	0.08–0.4	220 (3.6)	3.2–4.1	<0.001
Home support	80 (0.8)	3 (0.1)	0.07–0.2	77 (1.3)	0.09–1.6	<0.001
Palliative care	44 (0.4)	3 (0.1)	0.03–0.2	41 (0.7)	0.04–0.09	<0.001
Clinical variables						
High Risk Level	444 (4.5)	4 (0.1)	0.01–0.2	440 (7.3)	6.6–7.9	
Medium	1784 (18.1)	63 (1.6)	1.2–2.1	1721 (28.5)	27–30	<0.001
Low	7638 (77.4)	3763 (98.3)	97.8–98.6	3875 (64.2)	63–65	
Complexity weight *	6.7 (7.0)	2.9 (2.7)	2.8–3.0	9.1 (7.8)	8.9–9.3	<0.001
Chronic conditions *	2.5 (1.8)	1 (0.5)	0.8–1.2	3.5 (1.7)	3.4–3.6	<0.001
Polymedicated	1598 (16.2)	70 (1.8)	1.4–2.3	1528 (25.3)	24.2–26.4	<0.001

* Mean (standard deviation). CI: Confidence interval.

According to the AMG stratification, mean age increased as the risk level did, 58.6 years for low risk, 72.8 years for medium and 78.2 years for high. High-risk patients registered the worst functional status and the highest complexity (30.3 in high-risk patients vs. 12.5 in medium and 5.2 in low-risk patients) and rates of polypharmacy (79.8% of the high-risk patients vs. 44.1% of the medium-risk and 10.8% of the low-risk patients) (Table S2).

Regarding sex, women presented a higher average age (65.2 years vs. 62.1 years), higher prevalence of immobilization (5.6% vs. 3.4%), institutionalization (2.8% vs. 1.7%), need for caregivers (4.1% vs. 2.9%) and higher mean number of chronic diseases (3.6 vs. 3.4) and proportion of polymedication (27.6% vs. 21.3%). Relative to age groups, patients over 65 years had a higher prevalence of women (67% vs. 59.8%), immobilization (9.1% vs. 0.3%), need for institutionalization (4.6% vs. 0.1%) and caregivers (6.9% vs. 0.3%) and a higher mean number of chronic conditions (4.1 vs. 2.8) as well as more polymedication (48.9% vs. 1.1%) (Table S3).

The most prevalent chronic conditions within the population with multimorbidity were dyslipidemia (54.5%), hypertension (51.9%), obesity (22.9%), depression (17.7%) and osteoporosis (17.1%). In contrast, the most frequent diseases among the chronic population without multimorbidity were anxiety (17.7%), dyslipidemia (12.8%), asthma (11.6%), thyroid disorder (8.1%) and anemia (7.6%) (Table 2).

The most prevalent conditions among all risks were dyslipidemia and hypertension, followed by anxiety (30.0%) and thyroid disorder (21.2%) at the low risk level, obesity (26.9%) and diabetes (25.1%) at the medium risk level and dysrhythmias (43.6%) and neoplasia (37.3%) at the high risk level. (Table S4).

Table 2. Comorbidities in the total population with chronic conditions and with or without multimorbidity.

Comorbidities		Total	No Multimorbidity	95% CI	Multimorbidity	95% CI	p-Value
n (%)		9866 (100)	3830 (38.8)		6036 (61.2)		
Haematic comorbidity	Anemia	908 (9.2)	290 (7.6)	8.6–9.8	618 (10.2)	9.5–11.0	<0.001
	HIV	55 (0.6)	19 (0.5)	0.4–7.0	36 (0.6)	0.4–0.8	0.514
Digestive comorbidity	Cirrhosis	479 (4.9)	45 (1.2)	4.4–5.3	434 (7.2)	6.5–7.8	<0.001
	Inflammatory bowel disease	75 (0.8)	24 (0.6)	0.6–0.9	51 (0.8)	0.6–1.1	0.224
	Gastric ulcer	175 (1.8)	21 (0.5)	1.5–2.0	154 (2.6)	2.1–2.9	<0.001
	Chronic pancreatitis	8 (0.1)	1 (0.01)	0.01–0.2	7 (0.1)	0.03–0.2	0.162
	Cystic fibrosis	3 (0.03)	0 (0)	0.001–0.006	3 (0.01)	0.001–0.1	0.287
Ocular comorbidity	Glaucoma	395 (4.0)	39 (1.0)	3.6–4.4	356 (5.9)	5.3–6.45	<0.001
Cardio vascular comorbidity	Hypertension	3418 (34.6)	285 (7.4)	33.7–35.6	3133 (51.9)	50.6–53.2	<0.001
	Dysrhythmias	696 (7.1)	46 (1.2)	6.5–7.6	650 (10.8)	10.0–11.5	<0.001
	Chronic heart failure	240 (2.4)	2 (0.1)	2.1–2.7	238 (3.9)	3.4–4.4	<0.001
	Coronary disease	370 (3.8)	11 (0.3)	3.4–4.1	359 (5.9)	5.3–6.5	<0.001
	Valvular heart disease	196 (2.0)	11 (0.3)	1.7–2.3	185 (3.1)	2.4–3.5	<0.001
Musculo skeletal comorbidity	Osteoarthritis	1055 (10.7)	92 (2.4)	10.1–11.3	963 (16.0)	15.0–16.9	<0.001
	Osteoporosis	1113 (11.3)	79 (2.1)	10.6–11.9	1034 (17.1)	16.2–18.1	<0.001
	Arthritis	235 (2.4)	47 (1.2)	2.1–2.7	188 (3.1)	2.7–3.5	<0.001
	Lupus	5 (0.1)	1 (0.01)	0.06–0.9	4 (0.1)	0.001–0.013	0.655
	Vasculitis	27 (0.3)	1 (0.01)	0.1–0.5	26 (0.4)	0.3–0.6	<0.001
Neurological comorbidity	Dementia	213 (2.2)	13 (0.3)	1.8–2.5	200 (3.3)	2.9–3.8	<0.001
	Stroke	267 (2.7)	15 (0.4)	2.4–3.0	252 (4.2)	3.7–4.7	<0.001
	Parkinson	85 (0.9)	1 (0.01)	0.7–1.1	84 (1.4)	1.1–1.7	<0.001
	Epilepsy	187 (1.9)	60 (1.6)	1.6–2.2	127 (2.1)	1.7–2.5	0.056
	Multiple sclerosis	32 (0.3)	14 (0.4)	0.2–0.4	18 (0.3)	0.2–0.5	0.567
Psychiatric comorbidity	Alcohol abuse	407 (4.1)	55 (1.4)	3.7–4.5	352 (5.8)	5.2–6.4	<0.001
	Substance abuse	130 (1.3)	30 (0.8)	1.1–1.5	100 (1.7)	1.3–1.9	<0.001
	Anxiety	2345 (23.8)	678 (17.7)	22.9–24.6	1667 (27.6)	2.6–2.9	<0.001
	Depression	1251 (12.7)	181 (4.7)	12.0–13.3	1070 (17.7)	16.8–18.7	<0.001
	Bipolar illness	66 (0.7)	10 (0.3)	0.5–0.8	56 (0.9)	0.7–1.2	<0.001
	Psychotic disorder	74 (0.8)	9 (0.2)	0.6–0.9	65 (1.1)	0.8–1.3	<0.001
Respiratory comorbidity	COPD	389 (3.9)	22 (0.6)	3.5–4.3	367 (6.1)	5.5–6.7	<0.001
	Asthma	1044 (10.6)	444 (11.6)	10.0–11.2	600 (9.9)	9.2–10.7	0.009
Endocrine comorbidity	Dyslipidemia	3780 (38.3)	491 (12.8)	37.3–39.3	3289 (54.5)	53.2–55.7	<0.001
	Diabetes mellitus	1063 (10.8)	60 (1.6)	10.2–11.4	1003 (16.6)	15.7–17.6	<0.001
	Obesity	1625 (16.5)	241 (6.3)	15.7–17.2	1385 (22.9)	21.9–24.0	<0.001
	Thyroid disorder	1646 (16.7)	310 (8.1)	15.9–17.4	1336 (22.1)	21.1–23.2	<0.001
Renal comorbidity	Renal chronic failure	142 (1.4)	2 (0.1)	1.0–1.7	140 (2.3)	1.9–2.7	<0.001
	Repeat urinary tract infection	497 (5.0)	150 (3.9)	4.6–5.5	347 (5.7)	5.2–6.3	<0.001
Cancer comorbidity	Any cancer	481 (4.9)	54 (1.4)	4.4–5.3	427 (7.1)	76.4–7.7	<0.001
	Breast	74 (0.8)	12 (0.3)	0.5–0.9	62 (1.0)	0.8–1.3	<0.001
	Prostate	66 (0.7)	5 (0.1)	0.5–0.8	61 (1.0)	0.8–1.3	<0.001
	Skin	60 (0.6)	8 (0.2)	0.4–0.8	53 (0.9)	0.6–1.1	<0.001
	Colorectal	57 (0.6)	4 (0.1)	0.4–0.8	52 (0.9)	0.6–1.1	<0.001
	Bladder	35 (0.4)	1 (0.01)	0.2–0.6	34 (0.6)	0.4–0.7	<0.001
	Lung	34 (0.3)	1 (0.01)	0.2–0.4	33 (0.5)	0.3–0.7	<0.001
	Cervix	18 (0.2)	3 (0.1)	0.1–0.3	12 (0.2)	0.1–0.4	0.054
	Liver	7 (0.1)	2 (0.1)	0.01–0.2	5 (0.1)	0.01–0.2	0.578
	Gastric	8 (0.1)	0 (0)	0.01–0.2	8 (0.1)	0.04–0.2	0.024
	Pancreas	6 (0.1)	0 (0)	0.01–0.2	6 (0.1)	0.02–0.2	0.051
	Renal	12 (0.1)	0 (0)	0.01–0.2	12 (0.2)	0.1–0.3	0.006
	Endometrium	5 (0.1)	0 (0)	0.01–0.2	5 (0.1)	0.01–0.2	0.075
	Leukemia	27 (0.3)	2 (0.1)	0.2–0.4	25 (0.4)	0.2–0.6	<0.001
	Lymphoma	48 (0.5)	1 (0.01)	0.3–0.7	47 (0.8)	0.6–1.0	<0.001

CI: Confidence interval. COPD: Chronic obstructive pulmonary disease.

Some diseases were more prevalent among women, such as anxiety (31.6% vs. 20.7%), thyroid disorder (29.1% vs. 10.0%), osteoporosis (25.8% vs. 2%), depression (21.4% vs. 11.3%), anemia (12.2% vs. 6.8%), asthma (11.1% vs. 7.9%) and dementia (4% vs. 2.2%). In contrast, others were more prevalent among men: hypertension (57.1% vs. 48.9%), diabetes mellitus (21.9% vs. 13.6%), cirrhosis (9.3% vs. 6.0%), ischemic heart disease (10.1% vs. 3.5%), neoplasia (9.6% vs. 5.6%) and chronic obstructive pulmonary disease (COPD) (9.4% vs. 4.3%). Among patients aged >65 years, there was a higher prevalence of hypertension (72.1% vs. 31.1%), dyslipidemia (63.3% vs. 45.6%), osteoporosis (26.2% vs. 7.8%), diabetes (23.4% vs. 9.6%), neoplasia (9.5% vs. 4.5%), glaucoma (9.1% vs. 2.6%), dementia (6.3% and 0.2%) and stroke (6.8% vs. 1.5%), among other diseases. In contrast, alcohol abuse (8.1% vs. 3.6%), substance abuse (3.2% vs. 0.2%), anxiety (35.8% vs. 19.7%) and asthma (14.3% vs. 5.7%) were more prevalent in those $\leq$ 65 years of age. (Table S5).

Regarding the use of primary care services, the mean number of annual contacts in patients with multimorbidity was 14.9 and 6.3 in patients with only one chronic disease. The mean of contacts rose with the level of risk (9.8 in low risk, 21.5 in medium and 34.1 in high), and was higher in women than men (15.3 vs. 14.3) and in those >65 years old than in younger patients (19.6 vs. 10.1). The preferred contact form was face-to-face and health-related. Concerning the professional contacted, primary care doctors received a mean of 7.8 visits and primary care nurses 4.4, while the physiotherapists, midwives, dentists and social workers were contacted less frequently (Table 3, Tables S6 and S7).

Table 3. Annual primary care service utilization of the total population with chronic conditions and with or without multimorbidity.

Primary Care Contacts	Total	No Multimorbidity		Multimorbidity		p-Value
Mean (SD)	9866 (100%)	3830 (38.8%)	95% CI	6036 (61.2%)	95% CI	
Total Annual Contacts	11.5 (14.6)	6.3 (9.2)	6.0–6.6	14.9 (16.4)	14.5–15.3	<0.001
Type of contact						
Health-related	9.9 (12.8)	5.5 (8.0)	5.2–5.7	12.8 (14.3)	12.4–13.2	<0.001
Administrative	0.8 (3.3)	0.4 (1.9)	0.3–0.5	1.2 (3.9)	1.1–1.3	<0.001
Laboratory	0.7 (1.3)	0.4 (0.9)	0.3–0.5	0.9 (1.4)	0.9–1.0	<0.001
Form of contact						
Face-to-face	10.6 (12.5)	6.1 (8.5)	5.8–6.4	13.44 (13.8)	13.1–13.8	<0.001
Telephone	0.4 (2.2)	0.1 (0.9)	0.08–0.14	0.5 (2.7)	0.5–0.6	<0.001
Home visit	0.6 (3.9)	0.07 (1.0)	0.04–0.1	0.9 (4.9)	0.8–1.1	<0.001
Professional contacted						
Doctor	6.0 (7.1)	3.3 (4.8)	3.2–3.5	7.8 (7.7)	7.6–8.0	<0.001
Nurse	3.1 (7.0)	1.2 (3.7)	1.1–1.3	4.4 (8.2)	4.2–4.6	<0.001
Physiotherapist	0.3 (2.0)	0.2 (1.6)	0.1–0.3	0.3 (2.2)	0.3–0.4	0.064
Midwife	0.1 (7.2)	0.2 (1.0)	0.1–0.3	0.07 (0.4)	0.06–0.08	<0.001
Dentist	0.05 (0.4)	0.05 (0.4)	0.05–0.08	0.05 (0.4)	0.04–0.06	0.010
Social worker	0.07 (0.6)	0.02 (0.2)	0.01–0.03	0.1 (0.7)	0.09–0.12	<0.001

SD: Standard Deviation. CI: Confidence interval.

Sociodemographic and functional factors significantly associated with primary care utilization in patients with multimorbidity were age over 65 years (B Coefficient [BC] = 1.2; 95% Confidence Interval [CI] = 0.3–2.0), female sex (BC = 1.04; 95% CI = 0.3–1.8) and having a primary caregiver (BC = 8.7; 95% CI = 6.7–10.7). Clinical variables associated with greater utilization of primary care in patients with multimorbidity were complexity index (BC = 0.5; 95% CI = 0.4–0.6), risk level (BC = 2.3; 95% CI = 1.3–3.3), $\geq$ 3 chronic conditions (BC = 1.2; 95% CI = 0.4–2.0) and polymedication (BC = 5.1; 95% CI = 4.0–6.1). The chronic conditions causing a higher use of primary care were dysrhythmia (BC = 5.4; 95% CI = 4.2–6.7), dementia (BC = 4.8; 95% CI = 2.8–6.8) and diabetes (BC = 2.3; 95% CI = 1.3–3.3) (Table 4).

Table 4. Factors associated with the use of primary healthcare services in patients with multimorbidity.

Variables	B Coefficient	95% CI	p-Value
Primary caregiver	8.70	6.72–10.69	<0.001
Dysrhythmia	5.43	4.20–6.65	<0.001
Polymedicated	5.05	4.00–6.10	<0.001
Dementia	4.83	2.83–6.84	<0.001
Risk level	2.29	1.26–3.32	<0.001
Diabetes mellitus	2.27	1.28–3.27	<0.001
≥3 chronic diseases	1.20	0.37–2.04	0.005
Age > 65 years	1.15	0.30–2.01	0.008
Female sex	1.04	0.30–1.78	0.006
Complexity weight *	0.46	0.38–0.55	<0.001

Backward stepwise regression, $R^2 = 0.301$. * Continuous variable. CI: Confidence Interval.

4. Discussion

4.1. Main Findings

A total of 33.3% of the population from the healthcare area studied had multimorbidity. Their average age was almost 65 years old with a predominance of females, high complexity, medium and high risk levels, numerous chronic conditions and a greater need for assistance, care and polymedication compared to patients with only one chronic condition. The use of primary care services was notably high, mainly with family doctors, and was influenced by sociodemographic, functional and clinical factors.

4.2. Characteristics of the Population and Generalization of the Results

The prevalence of multimorbidity was 33.3%, close to the 37.2% described worldwide in a recent systematic review and meta-analysis [2], where regional estimates varied depending on the population, age group, and chronic conditions or multimorbidity definition considered [2,4]. As expected, the population with multimorbidity studied had an advanced mean age [12–20] and almost two-thirds were women, coinciding with the predominance of this sex within multimorbid populations described in other series from different regions around the world [13,14,17–19]. Patients with multimorbidity had higher levels of immobility, institutionalization and need for caregivers due to their functional impairment caused by their multiple chronic conditions and complexity, as observed in other populations with multimorbidity [16,20–23]. The most frequent chronic conditions were similar to other series of patients with multimorbidity across the globe [10,12,14–17,19–21,24], predominately cardiovascular, osteoarticular, psychiatric and neoplasms.

Our results coincided with the populations with multimorbidity described by Rizza et al. [13], Linden et al. [14] and Ibarra-Castillo et al. [19] identifying a higher prevalence of chronic diseases in women; the proportion of women decreased in the high risk level, but was still more representative than men. In line with a review focusing on the interplay between multimorbidity and functional impairment [23], high-risk patients presented more functional impairment and immobility and required more frequent caregivers and palliative care. Low-risk multimorbid patients often had two mild chronic conditions, while medium-risk patients normally had more than four diseases and were similar in frequencies and characteristics to pluripathological patients [16], whereas high-risk patients could be compared to complex chronic patients with more functional and fragile deterioration [12]. The most frequent diseases in high- and medium-risk patients were hypertension, diabetes, neoplasms, obesity and heart failure, while low-risk patients predominantly had dyslipidemia, anxiety and thyroid disorders, as observed in other adult populations with multimorbidity [12,13]. Polypharmacy was increased in high-risk patients, as a higher prescription of medication is frequently associated with higher complexity and greater comorbidities [16,25].

Women were older and had greater immobility, with an almost doubled need for care, more chronic diseases and more polypharmacy than men, as described previously [14,20,26]. Anxiety, thyroid disorder, osteoporosis, depression, anemia and dementia predominated in women, while hypertension, cirrhosis, COPD, ischemic heart disease and neoplasia predominated in men, in line with other studies analyzing populations with multimorbidity by sex [14,21,26].

Regarding age, patients with multimorbidity over 65 years had a female predominance, given that women have a longer lifespan [14,20,26]. Older patients presented with more immobilization, greater needs of care, and higher quantity and severity of chronic conditions, as observed by other authors [14,15,23,26]. Predominant chronic conditions in the elderly were hypertension, osteoporosis, diabetes, neoplasia, glaucoma, dementia and stroke, as described in other aged populations [15,21,26]. Almost half of the elderly were polymedicated, in contrast to 1% of younger patients, explained because multimorbidity, which increases with age, increases complications and health adverse events, so more medication is needed to control concomitant chronic diseases [25].

4.3. Use of Primary Healthcare Services

A remarkably high number of contacts with the primary care system was observed in the patients with multimorbidity, supporting the literature [10,12,17,18,24,26–28] and the fact that multimorbidity has been estimated to account for 78% of all primary care consultations [29]. Multimorbidity patients tripled the average primary care contacts registered by the general population of Madrid the previous year [30], being this threefold difference in accordance with data reported by other studies [17,24,27]. The family doctor was the most contacted type of professional, pursuant to the gatekeeping system of the Spanish National Health System [11] and with the mean annual contacts registered with this professional by Cassell et al. [17], Bähler et al. [18] and Soley-Bori et al. [27]. The number of contacts with a nurse was lower than expected according to Madrid's model of care for addressing chronicity, which promotes a key role of nurses prioritizing most of the follow-up and care of the patients, while doctors should only intervene when medical care is needed or in situations of greater complexity [7]. Following this strategy, the role of the social worker was also expected to be higher. Regardless, telephone contacts and home visits should be increased in the context of care for multimorbidity patients [18,27], as these were truly low.

Every contact with primary care in multimorbidity patients increased according to the risk level [28]. The mean number of contacts with family doctors was higher among women, as they often report a worse perceived health status and have more minor affective disorders that can cause more doctor consultations [21]. In contrast, primary care nurse consultations were higher among men, perhaps due to less self-care capacity, as it is usually described among elderly men [31]. It is noteworthy how aged patients with multimorbidity patients had a nearly two-fold amount of total contact with primary care physicians compared to younger patients, since they usually have more complexity and comorbidities [18,24,28].

The variable with the greatest impact on the use of primary care services was having a primary caregiver, since patients who require this assistance often present with severe chronic diseases and functional and cognitive limitations and disabilities impeding them from getting healthcare services by themselves; thus, caregivers provide them assistance and facilitate access to healthcare services and transitions between healthcare professionals [32]. Being polymedicated was also highly associated with the utilization of healthcare services as polypharmacy is related to suffering a greater number of diseases with greater severity, mostly leading to higher use of services due to frequent dose adjustments by primary care professionals or due to errors in medication intake, adverse effects or interactions between drugs [25,27,28]. In the same way, primary care utilization was influenced by the AMG complexity degree, high risk level and having numerous chronic conditions, as observed in other studies with complex patients or with multimorbidity [12,18,26,28]. The association between advanced age in patients with multimorbidity and the use of services was evident [18–20,24,26,28]. As well, the female sex was significantly linked to higher healthcare utilization, probably because as women have a longer life expectancy they often suffer from a worse health status requiring more visits to the primary care system [13,14,26]; in addition, women typically evaluate their health and health-related outcomes worse than males [21]. Finally, the diseases dysrhythmia, diabetes and dementia were correlated with increased primary care utilization because these pathologies require continuous monitoring by primary care professionals, involving routine adjustment of medication dosage and frequent control of symptoms [33,34].

4.4. Limitations

The use of secondary data sources could cause possible biases of information linked to the variability in the way the different health professionals registered the diseases. Nevertheless, the use of clinical–administrative sources for epidemiological studies is widespread, providing real-world data and facilitating work with almost all individuals and not with partial samples, minimizing possible selection and memory biases. There could be patients not represented in the total population of the basic healthcare area if they had private insurance, but this is unlikely to bias the results because Madrid public health insurance covers almost the entire population [11].

Morbidity groupers have raised doubts about their transparency and their calculations of complexity, and commonly do not consider socioeconomic status, frailty or disability, need for care, clinical values or prognostic rating scales. AMG has overcome these problems and has proven its validity compared to other groupers [35]. Lastly, some chronic diseases may have not been considered by the AMG, which only takes into account the ones described by the Community of Madrid Strategy of Care for Patients with Chronic Diseases [7]; likewise, this problem affects any study with chronic diseases since no universal definition has been established.

Although the data were extracted from a unique healthcare area, all the results are representative of the Madrid population with chronic diseases and multimorbidity and could be extrapolated to the rest of the Spanish territory and outside Spain, since this healthcare area serves a widely heterogeneous group of people, including patients of different conditions and nationalities. Additionally, our results showed similar trends to the ones observed in other studies conducted around the world.

The COVID-19 pandemic introduced great challenges in the organization of health centers. Work systems and relationship models with patients may have experienced an increase in non-face-to-face contact. For that reason, the mean number of telephone contacts is likely to be higher nowadays, as this global event has shown that telephonic consultations are a useful tool to support the traditional care model. Nevertheless, despite that the data may seem outdated, the results obtained regarding the utilization of primary care services by the Madrid population described for the year of our study [36] are very close in numbers to those stated in the last Annual Report of Madrid Health Service [37]. Therefore, the healthcare utilization findings presented in this study depict the current reality and are of great importance and usefulness.

4.5. Implications

Patients with multimorbidity create a high care burden for the primary care system. These patients require the development of personalized management approaches made by primary care professionals, with the aim of improving the quality and continuity of care, as well as optimizing the healthcare services offered and reducing the costs derived from fragmented care [3,7]. For designing novel healthcare strategies, it is necessary to thoroughly characterize this population.

All the characteristics and use of primary care services in the multimorbid population described in this study provide valuable information that will help researchers, primary care professionals and healthcare policymakers. Understanding the findings depicted will facilitate the provision of holistic and evidence-based care and allocation of resources, focusing on the real situation and existing needs of patients with multimorbidity with the purpose of improving the quality and life expectancy of patients while also optimizing the utilization of primary care services, thereby reducing important healthcare costs and boosting the sustainability of healthcare systems [3,4,8]. Additionally, morbidity groupers such as the novel AMG support primary care professionals in identifying these patients and developing individualized interventions adapted to multimorbidity patient care needs, prioritizing those with higher risk and complexity [9,10], as recommended in the Madrid Care Strategy for people with chronic diseases [7].

5. Conclusions

Multimorbidity patients represent an important percentage of the population. They are older, with a female predominance and important needs of care, suffering from several comorbidities and polypharmacy, a situation that worsens with the AMG's level of risk and complexity. The utilization of primary care services is extremely high, mostly directed to family doctors and mainly associated with sociodemographic factors such as old age and female sex, functional factors such as having a primary caregiver, and clinical factors such as complexity index, high risk level, the presence of numerous chronic diseases and polymedication. This study provides novel data on risk levels by the novel AMG grouper in multimorbidity patients, as well as characterizes the utilization of health services and needs of care. Understanding these valuable real-world data could profoundly help primary care professionals and policymakers to improve coordination between healthcare professionals and allocation of services to optimize multimorbidity management and ensure a better quality of life for patients as well as to reduce costs derived from their extensive health service utilization.

Supplementary Materials: The following supporting information can be downloaded at: https://www.mdpi.com/article/10.3390/healthcare12020270/s1, Table S1: Types of chronic diseases considered by the Adjusted Morbidity Group (AMG) in the Community of Madrid at the time of data extraction; Table S2: Sociodemographic, functional and clinical characteristics of the patients with multimorbidity by risk level according to Adjusted Morbidity Groups; Table S3: Sociodemographic, functional and clinical characteristics of the patients with multimorbidity by sex and age group; Table S4: Comorbidities of the patients with multimorbidity by risk level according to Adjusted Morbidity Groups; Table S5: Comorbidities of the patients with multimorbidity by sex and age group; Table S6: Annual primary care services utilization in patients with multimorbidity by risk level according to Adjusted Morbidity Groups; Table S7: Annual primary care services utilization in patients with multimorbidity by sex and age group.

Author Contributions: Conceptualization, J.B.-C. and M.T.B.-M.; methodology, J.B.-C., A.C.-R., B.B.-S. and M.T.B.-M.; software, J.B.-C.; validation, J.B.-C., A.C.-R., B.B.-S. and M.T.B.-M.; formal analysis, J.B.-C., A.C.-R., B.B.-S. and M.T.B.-M.; investigation, J.B.-C., A.C.-R., B.B.-S. and M.T.B.-M.; resources, J.B.-C.; data curation, J.B.-C., A.C.-R., B.B.-S. and M.T.B.-M.; writing—original draft preparation, J.B.-C., A.C.-R., B.B.-S., M.T.B.-M. and C.R.-Z.; writing—review and editing, J.B.-C., A.C.-R., B.B.-S., M.T.B.-M. and C.R.-Z.; visualization, J.B.-C., A.C.-R., B.B.-S., M.T.B.-M. and C.R.-Z.; supervision, J.B.-C.; project administration, J.B.-C.; funding acquisition, J.B.-C. All authors have read and agreed to the published version of the manuscript.

Funding: This project received a grant for English editing and for publication from the Foundation for Biosanitary Research and Innovation in Primary Care (FIIBAP) through its funding policy for scientific publications for the second semester of 2023.

Institutional Review Board Statement: This study was conducted according to the guidelines of the Declaration of Helsinki, and approved by the Hospital Universitario La Princesa Drug Research Ethics Committee (approval number 10/17, protocol number 3105, approval date 25 May 2017) and obtained a favorable report from the Local Research Commission of the Primary Care Management of the Community of Madrid (protocol number 08/17-C, approval date 9 May 2017). All methods were performed in accordance with the relevant guidelines and regulations.

Informed Consent Statement: Patient consent was waived because this study is retrospective and does not contain any individual personal data since the data was obtained from a secondary database with anonymized and dissociated information.

Data Availability Statement: The datasets generated and analyzed during the current study are not publicly available because they belong to the Madrid Health Service, but they are available from the corresponding author on reasonable request.

Acknowledgments: We would like to thank the Research Unit of the Primary Care Management of Madrid for their methodological support.

Conflicts of Interest: The authors declare no conflict of interest.

References

1. Skou, S.T.; Mair, F.S.; Fortin, M.; Guthrie, B.; Nunes, B.P.; Miranda, J.J.; Boyd, C.M.; Pati, S.; Mtenga, S.; Smith, S.M. Multimorbidity. *Nat. Rev. Dis. Primers* **2022**, *8*, 48. [CrossRef] [PubMed]
2. Chowdhury, S.R.; Chandra Das, D.; Sunna, T.C.; Beyene, J.; Hossain, A. Global and Regional Prevalence of Multimorbidity in the Adult Population in Community Settings: A Systematic Review and Meta-Analysis. *EClinicalMedicine* **2023**, *57*, 101860. [CrossRef] [PubMed]
3. Aramrat, C.; Choksomngam, Y.; Jiraporncharoen, W.; Wiwatkunupakarn, N.; Pinyopornpanish, K.; Mallinson, P.A.C.; Kinra, S.; Angkurawaranon, C. Advancing Multimorbidity Management in Primary Care: A Narrative Review. *Prim. Health Care Res. Dev.* **2022**, *23*, e36. [CrossRef]
4. Ho, I.S.-S.; Azcoaga-Lorenzo, A.; Akbari, A.; Black, C.; Davies, J.; Hodgins, P.; Khunti, K.; Kadam, U.; Lyons, R.A.; McCowan, C.; et al. Examining Variation in the Measurement of Multimorbidity in Research: A Systematic Review of 566 Studies. *Lancet Public Health* **2021**, *6*, e587–e597. [CrossRef] [PubMed]
5. Ansah, J.P.; Chiu, C.-T. Projecting the Chronic Disease Burden among the Adult Population in the United States Using a Multi-State Population Model. *Front. Public Health* **2022**, *10*, 1082183. [CrossRef] [PubMed]
6. Pearson-Stuttard, J.; Ezzati, M.; Gregg, E.W. Multimorbidity-a Defining Challenge for Health Systems. *Lancet Public Health* **2019**, *4*, e599–e600. [CrossRef] [PubMed]
7. Madrid Health Service. *Care Strategy for People with Chronic Diseases in the Community of Madrid*; Madrid Health Service: Madrid, Spain, 2013. Available online: https://www.madrid.org/bvirtual/BVCM017570.pdf (accessed on 29 August 2023).
8. Mora, J.; Iturralde, M.D.; Prieto, L.; Domingo, C.; Gagnon, M.-P.; Martínez-Carazo, C.; March, A.G.; De Massari, D.; Martí, T.; Nalin, M.; et al. Key Aspects Related to Implementation of Risk Stratification in Health Care Systems-the ASSEHS Study. *BMC Health Serv. Res.* **2017**, *17*, 331. [CrossRef] [PubMed]
9. Monterde, D.; Vela, E.; Clèries, M. Adjusted morbidity groups: A new multiple morbidity measurement of use in Primary Care. *Aten. Primaria* **2016**, *48*, 674–682. [CrossRef]
10. Monterde, D.; Vela, E.; Clèries, M.; Garcia-Eroles, L.; Roca, J.; Pérez-Sust, P. Multimorbidity as a Predictor of Health Service Utilization in Primary Care: A Registry-Based Study of the Catalan Population. *BMC Fam. Pract.* **2020**, *21*, 39. [CrossRef]
11. Fernández-Pérez, Á.; Jiménez-Rubio, D.; Robone, S. Freedom of Choice and Health Services' Performance: Evidence from a National Health System. *Health Policy* **2022**, *126*, 1283–1290. [CrossRef]
12. Figueroa, J.F.; Papanicolas, I.; Riley, K.; Abiona, O.; Arvin, M.; Atsma, F.; Bernal-Delgado, E.; Bowden, N.; Blankart, C.R.; Deeny, S.; et al. International Comparison of Health Spending and Utilization among People with Complex Multimorbidity. *Health Serv. Res.* **2021**, *56* (Suppl. S3), 1317–1334. [CrossRef] [PubMed]
13. Rizza, A.; Kaplan, V.; Senn, O.; Rosemann, T.; Bhend, H.; Tandjung, R. Age- and Gender-Related Prevalence of Multimorbidity in Primary Care: The Swiss Fire Project. *BMC Fam. Pract.* **2012**, *13*, 113. [CrossRef]
14. Linden, M.; Linden, U.; Goretzko, D.; Gensichen, J. Prevalence and Pattern of Acute and Chronic Multimorbidity across All Body Systems and Age Groups in Primary Health Care. *Sci. Rep.* **2022**, *12*, 272. [CrossRef] [PubMed]
15. Excoffier, S.; Herzig, L.; N'Goran, A.A.; Déruaz-Luyet, A.; Haller, D.M. Prevalence of Multimorbidity in General Practice: A Cross-Sectional Study within the Swiss Sentinel Surveillance System (Sentinella). *BMJ Open* **2018**, *8*, e019616. [CrossRef] [PubMed]
16. Martín Lesende, I.; Mendibil Crespo, L.I.; Castaño Manzanares, S.; Otter, A.-S.D.; Garaizar Bilbao, I.; Pisón Rodríguez, J.; Negrete Pérez, I.; Sarduy Azcoaga, I.; de la Rua Fernández, M.J. Functional Decline and Associated Factors in Patients with Multimorbidity at 8 Months of Follow-up in Primary Care: The Functionality in Pluripathological Patients (FUNCIPLUR) Longitudinal Descriptive Study. *BMJ Open* **2018**, *8*, e022377. [CrossRef] [PubMed]
17. Cassell, A.; Edwards, D.; Harshfield, A.; Rhodes, K.; Brimicombe, J.; Payne, R.; Griffin, S. The Epidemiology of Multimorbidity in Primary Care: A Retrospective Cohort Study. *Br. J. Gen. Pract. J. R. Coll. Gen. Pract.* **2018**, *68*, e245–e251. [CrossRef]
18. Bähler, C.; Huber, C.A.; Brüngger, B.; Reich, O. Multimorbidity, Health Care Utilization and Costs in an Elderly Community-Dwelling Population: A Claims Data Based Observational Study. *BMC Health Serv. Res.* **2015**, *15*, 23. [CrossRef]
19. Ibarra-Castillo, C.; Guisado-Clavero, M.; Violan-Fors, C.; Pons-Vigués, M.; López-Jiménez, T.; Roso-Llorach, A. Survival in Relation to Multimorbidity Patterns in Older Adults in Primary Care in Barcelona, Spain (2010–2014): A Longitudinal Study Based on Electronic Health Records. *J. Epidemiol. Community Health* **2018**, *72*, 185–192. [CrossRef]
20. Pascual-de la Pisa, B.; Cuberos-Sánchez, C.; Marquez-Calzada, C.; Garcia-Lozano, M.; Pardo-Alvarez, J.; Ollero-Baturone, M. Mortality and associated factors of patients with complex chronic diseases in rural and social transformation areas in Andalusia. *Med. Fam. Semer.* **2020**, *46*, 115–124. [CrossRef]

21. Violan, C.; Foguet-Boreu, Q.; Flores-Mateo, G.; Salisbury, C.; Blom, J.; Freitag, M.; Glynn, L.; Muth, C.; Valderas, J.M. Prevalence, Determinants and Patterns of Multimorbidity in Primary Care: A Systematic Review of Observational Studies. *PLoS ONE* **2014**, *9*, e102149. [CrossRef]
22. Prazeres, F.; Santiago, L. Prevalence of Multimorbidity in the Adult Population Attending Primary Care in Portugal: A Cross-Sectional Study. *BMJ Open* **2015**, *5*, e009287. [CrossRef] [PubMed]
23. Calderón-Larrañaga, A.; Vetrano, D.L.; Ferrucci, L.; Mercer, S.W.; Marengoni, A.; Onder, G.; Eriksdotter, M.; Fratiglioni, L. Multimorbidity and Functional Impairment-Bidirectional Interplay, Synergistic Effects and Common Pathways. *J. Intern. Med.* **2019**, *285*, 255–271. [CrossRef] [PubMed]
24. Quinaz Romana, G.; Kislaya, I.; Cunha Gonçalves, S.; Salvador, M.R.; Nunes, B.; Matias Dias, C. Healthcare Use in Patients with Multimorbidity. *Eur. J. Public Health* **2020**, *30*, 16–22. [CrossRef] [PubMed]
25. Khezrian, M.; McNeil, C.J.; Murray, A.D.; Myint, P.K. An Overview of Prevalence, Determinants and Health Outcomes of Polypharmacy. *Ther. Adv. Drug Saf.* **2020**, *11*, 2042098620933741. [CrossRef] [PubMed]
26. Foguet-Boreu, Q.; Violan, C.; Roso-Llorach, A.; Rodriguez-Blanco, T.; Pons-Vigués, M.; Muñoz-Pérez, M.A.; Pujol-Ribera, E.; Valderas, J.M. Impact of Multimorbidity: Acute Morbidity, Area of Residency and Use of Health Services across the Life Span in a Region of South Europe. *BMC Fam. Pract.* **2014**, *15*, 55. [CrossRef] [PubMed]
27. Soley-Bori, M.; Bisquera, A.; Ashworth, M.; Wang, Y.; Durbaba, S.; Dodhia, H.; Fox-Rushby, J. Identifying Multimorbidity Clusters with the Highest Primary Care Use: 15 Years of Evidence from a Multi-Ethnic Metropolitan Population. *Br. J. Gen. Pract. J. R. Coll. Gen. Pract.* **2022**, *72*, e190–e198. [CrossRef] [PubMed]
28. Heins, M.; Korevaar, J.; Schellevis, F.; Rijken, M. Identifying Multimorbid Patients with High Care Needs—A Study Based on Electronic Medical Record Data. *Eur. J. Gen. Pract.* **2020**, *26*, 189–195. [CrossRef]
29. Salisbury, C.; Johnson, L.; Purdy, S.; Valderas, J.M.; Montgomery, A.A. Epidemiology and Impact of Multimorbidity in Primary Care: A Retrospective Cohort Study. *Br. J. Gen. Pract.* **2011**, *61*, e12–e21. [CrossRef]
30. Madrid Health Service. *Annual Report of Madrid Health Service 2014*; Madrid Health Service: Madrid, Spain, 2015. Available online: https://gestiona3.madrid.org/bvirtual/BVCM017836.pdf (accessed on 16 October 2023).
31. Mei, J.; Tian, Y.; Chai, X.; Fan, X. Gender Differences in Self-Care Maintenance and Its Associations among Patients with Chronic Heart Failure. *Int. J. Nurs. Sci.* **2019**, *6*, 58–64. [CrossRef]
32. Fortinsky, R.H. Family Caregiver Assessment in Primary Care: How to Strengthen the HealthCare Triad? *J. Am. Geriatr. Soc.* **2021**, *69*, 286–288. [CrossRef]
33. Lee, S.-R.; Ahn, H.-J.; Choi, E.-K.; Lee, S.-W.; Han, K.-D.; Oh, S.; Lip, G.Y.H. Improved Prognosis with Integrated Care Management Including Early Rhythm Control and Healthy Lifestyle Modification in Patients with Concurrent Atrial Fibrillation and Diabetes Mellitus: A Nationwide Cohort Study. *Cardiovasc. Diabetol.* **2023**, *22*, 18. [CrossRef] [PubMed]
34. Bergman, H.; Borson, S.; Jessen, F.; Krolak-Salmon, P.; Pirani, A.; Rasmussen, J.; Rodrigo, J.; Taddeo, D. Dementia and Comorbidities in Primary Care: A Scoping Review. *BMC Prim. Care* **2023**, *24*, 277. [CrossRef] [PubMed]
35. Arias-López, C.; Rodrigo Val, M.P.; Casaña Fernández, L.; Salvador Sánchez, L.; Dorado Díaz, A.; Estupiñán Ramírez, M. Validity of predictive power of the Adjusted Morbidity Groups (AMG) with respect to others population stratification tools. *Rev. Esp. Salud Publica* **2020**, *94*, e202007079. [PubMed]
36. Madrid Health Service. *Annual Report of the Madrid Health Service 2015*; Madrid Health Service: Madrid, Spain, 2016. Available online: http://www.madrid.org/bvirtual/BVCM017932.pdf (accessed on 1 November 2023).
37. Madrid Health Service. *Annual Report of Madrid Health Service 2022*; Madrid Health Service: Madrid, Spain, 2023. Available online: https://gestiona3.madrid.org/bvirtual/BVCM050988.pdf (accessed on 1 November 2023).

Disclaimer/Publisher's Note: The statements, opinions and data contained in all publications are solely those of the individual author(s) and contributor(s) and not of MDPI and/or the editor(s). MDPI and/or the editor(s) disclaim responsibility for any injury to people or property resulting from any ideas, methods, instructions or products referred to in the content.

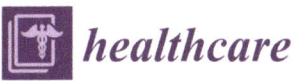

Article

Poverty Reduction Effects of Medical Insurance on Middle-Aged and Elderly Families under the Goal of Common Prosperity in China

Linhong Chen [1] and Xiaocang Xu [2,*]

[1] School of Marxism, Chongqing Technology and Business University, Chongqing 400067, China
[2] School of Economics and Management, Huzhou University, Huzhou 313000, China
* Correspondence: 03122@zjhu.edu.cn

Abstract: Eliminating poverty due to illness is an important way for China to pursue common prosperity. The high medical expenditure caused by the aging population has brought severe challenges to governments and families of all countries, especially in China, where the entire population has just been lifted out of poverty in 2020 and then hit by COVID-19. How to prevent the possible return of poor boundary families to poverty in China has become a difficult research topic. Based on the latest data from the China Health and Retirement Longitudinal Survey, this paper discusses the poverty reduction effect of medical insurance on middle-aged and elderly families from the absolute index and relative index. Medical insurance had a poverty reduction effect on middle-aged and elderly families, especially the poor boundary families. For example, people who participated in medical insurance reduced their financial burden by 2.36% for middle-aged and older families compared to people who did not participate in medical insurance. Furthermore, the poverty reduction effect had heterogeneity in gender and age. This research brings some policy implications. For example, the government should give more protection to vulnerable groups such as the elderly and low-income families and improve the fairness and effectiveness of the medical insurance system.

Keywords: common prosperity; poverty reduction effect; medical insurance; relative index; family medical financial burden

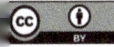

1. Introduction

China has entered a stage of population aging, with the proportion of people aged 65 and above in the total population rising from 10.5% in 2015 to 13.5% in 2020. The dependency ratio of the elderly has also soared from 37% in 2015 to 45.9% in 2020, and about 190 million of them suffer from chronic diseases. This poses a serious challenge to both the government and families' medical expenditure burden (China Health Statistical Yearbook, 2021). From 2015 to 2020, the proportion of total medical expenditure in GDP increased from 5.95% to 7.1%, the per capita medical expenditure for outpatients increased from CNY 233.9 to CNY 324.4, and the per capita medical expenditure for inpatients increased from CNY 8268.1 to CNY 10,619.2 (Figure 1). The rapid growth of medical expenditure puts a heavy economic burden on the whole of society [1]. At the same time, since the establishment of the basic medical insurance system in 1998, China has formed a basic pattern of social medical insurance, with the main insurance as the primary and commercial medical insurance as the auxiliary, but there are still some limitations such as system decentralization and system fairness to be improved. In addition, moral hazards, information asymmetry, and other issues, as well as public health emergencies such as COVID-19, have impacted the development of the health service system in China.

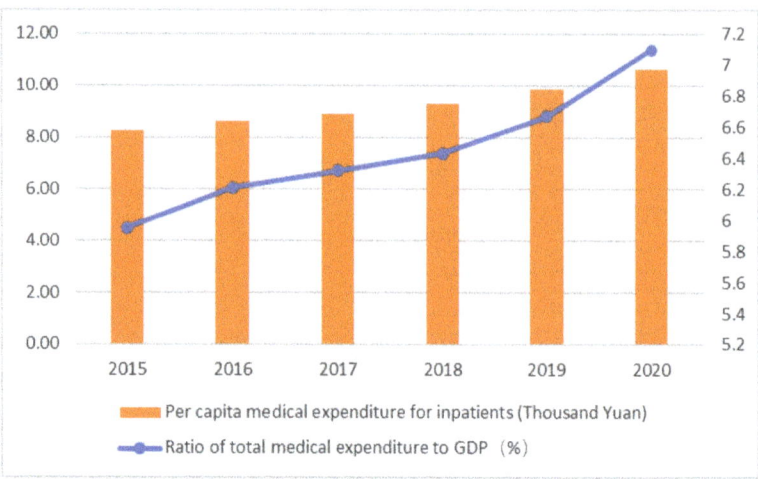

Figure 1. Burden of medical expenditure in China from 2015 to 2020. Source: China Health Statistical Yearbook 2021.

Scholars generally believe that medical insurance can cause the growth of the utilization rate of health services to varying degrees and improve the health status of residents [2,3]. The research on the impact of medical insurance on medical expenditure mainly focuses on the following four aspects.

First, medical insurance can improve the level of medical consumption and reduce the medical economic burden. Medical insurance subsidizes residents' medical expenditures so that residents can enjoy the same or even better health services with lower out-of-pocket medical expenses, which can reduce the burden of residents' medical expenditures. Zang and Zhang (2019) [4] believe that there is a substitution effect between medical insurance and family intergenerational economic support. Jung and Liu (2015) [5] and Kang and Barner (2017) [6] obtained two different opinions on the provision of medical insurance, i.e., the level of out-of-pocket medical expenditures decreases and there is no difference, respectively, while Choi et al. (2018) [7] and Feng et al. (2020) [8] confirmed the positive role of long-term care insurance. Furthermore, the higher the level of medical insurance, the more obvious its positive effect on medical expenditure [9,10].

Second, medical insurance can reduce the incidence of catastrophic medical expenditures and crowd out preventive saving behavior, which further effectively prevents the generation of "poverty caused by illness" [11,12]. Zhu and Shi (2016) [13] used heckprobit models to empirically study the impact of floating population participation in basic medical insurance on catastrophic medical expenditures and proposed that medical insurance with a higher reimbursement ratio of floating population participation is less prone to catastrophic medical expenditures.

Third, medical insurance shows heterogeneity in different income groups and the fairness of the system needs to be improved. Specifically, the medical expenditure effect of medical insurance on low-income groups is not obvious, but it can promote the medical expenditure of middle and high-income groups [14,15]. Yu et al. (2018) [16] found that the social medical insurance system did not have a significant positive impact on the medical consumption and health status of vulnerable elderly groups whereas Chen et al. (2019) [17] and Kwon et al. (2015) [18] found that medical insurance did not significantly reduce the medical expenditure of ordinary people and that the out-of-pocket medical expenditures of the rich are actually reduced more.

Fourth, the positive effect of medical insurance on medical expenditure is limited by information asymmetry, moral hazard, and other factors [19,20]. Similarly, as medical insurance lowers the threshold of access to health services, residents can enjoy health services at a lower cost, which to a certain extent leads to the abuse of health services such as excessive medical treatment, resulting in the unreasonable growth of medical expenditure [21]. Ren et al. (2014) [22] and Zhao et al. (2021) [23] found that elderly people with poor health status were more inclined to participate in medical insurance, and that the frequency of participating in physical exercise decreased significantly after obtaining insurance, which confirmed the existence of adverse selection and moral hazard in medical insurance.

In summary, the academia on the poverty reduction effect of medical insurance on elderly families has reached a basic consensus: medical insurance can reduce the medical expenditure burden of the government and the family and reduce the incidence rate of catastrophic health expenditure, which reduces the risk of family poverty due to illness. However, the actual effect of the poverty reduction effect is debated, due to imbalanced outpatient-hospitalization problems caused by information asymmetry and moral hazard, and the heterogeneity between different genders and ages and especially between high-income and low-income families. These problems reserve certain research space and hold value in this paper. Therefore, this paper raises the research question, what are the characteristics of the poverty reduction effect of medical insurance on middle-aged and elderly families under the background of China's special national conditions? In order to answer this question, this paper selects the latest data from the China Health and Retirement Longitudinal Survey (CHARLS) and uses the absolute index (total medical expenditure) and relative index (proportion of medical expenditure in per capita annual income) to discuss the poverty reduction effect of medical insurance on middle-aged and elderly families and its characteristics regarding urban-rural, gender, and age differences.

2. Materials and Methods

2.1. Theoretical Analysis

The poverty reduction effect of medical insurance on middle-aged and elderly families is mainly through influencing individual health and the utilization of health services.

(1) Individual health. Medical insurance affects individual health status and medical expenditure through daily health behavior factors. On the one hand, medical insurance can remind residents to pay attention to their health status and improve their awareness of health care. On the other hand, the existence of medical insurance can reduce the economic cost of bad health behaviors to a certain extent. Moral hazards may encourage more bad health behaviors and bring a negative impact on residents' health status. Cao and Tan (2022) [24] used the CHARLS data to empirically conclude that the frequency of physical examination of middle-aged and elderly people participating in medical insurance has decreased, which makes the health effect of medical insurance discounted due to moral hazard.

(2) Use of health services. Medical insurance reduces the relative price and access threshold of health services through the subsidy of medical expenditures, releasing the potential medical demand that had been restrained by economic factors, giving citizens more opportunities to improve their health status through health services, and at the same time increasing the consumption level of health services. Xu and Gu (2022) [25] used the differential-difference model and found that the critical illness insurance system could increase the hospitalization probability of middle-aged and elderly residents by 1.03%.

2.2. Variable Selection

Based on the above theoretical basis and research assumptions, this paper constructed the following variable system and analyzed the poverty reduction effect of medical insurance on middle-aged and elderly families by discussing the impact of medical insurance on their health status and medical expenditure.

2.2.1. Explained Variables: Total Medical Expenditure (Absolute Index) and Family Medical Economic Pressure (Relative Index)

Most existing research tends to assess the utilization of health services from the use frequency and consumption expenditure of health services, such as outpatient expenditure, hospitalization expenditure, or total medical expenditure, within a certain period. This paper selects medical expenditure and medical economic burden for the family as explained variables. The total medical expenditure (absolute index) is the sum of the recent outpatients' outlays and inpatients' outlays in the past year, and the family medical economic burden (relative index) is the proportion of medical expenditure in the per capita annual income of middle-aged and elderly families.

2.2.2. Main Explanatory Variable: Medical Insurance

Whether to participate in medical insurance (including medical insurance for urban and rural residents, medical insurance for urban residents, and new rural cooperative medical insurance) is selected as the core explanatory variable. In our paper, if the respondent has participated in medical insurance, the value assigned is 1, otherwise, the value assigned is 0. The corresponding title for the questionnaire is "Do you currently participate in the following medical insurance?".

2.2.3. Other Explanatory Variables

Medical expenditure is not only affected by the characteristics of medical insurance but is also affected by many other factors, including health status. When selecting other explanatory variables, this study selected other explanatory variables from four aspects: environmental factors, personal characteristics, health behaviors, and health outcomes. Take the nominal variables as an example: 1 for males and 0 for females in the Gender value; unmarried (never married or cohabitation) or divorced (no longer married, separated as a spouse, divorced, or widowed) is "0", and married is "1" in the Marital status value, and so on. Additionally, in terms of the Ordinal variables, the self-rated health status was given as "0" for "very poor" and "poor", "1" for "fair", and "2" for "good" and "very good". Weekly activity level was assigned with inactive as "0", low-intensity physical activity as "1", moderate-intensity physical activity as "2", and high-intensity physical activity as "3".

2.3. Empirical Tools

The medical expenditure data in CHARLS presented an obviously skewed distribution. If OLS regression is performed directly, it often leads to selective bias and other endogenous problems. Therefore, the two-part model and Heckman sample selection model are used in this paper to explore the impact of medical insurance on the medical expenditure of middle-aged and elderly people. First, the logarithm of medical expenditure data is processed, and then the two-part model and sample Heckman selection model are chosen, to deal with possible sample selection bias and selective bias problem, respectively, at the same time to test each other between the two models to determine if their conclusions are consistent; the empirical results are robust.

Firstly, the two-part model is used to deal with endogeneity problems caused by medical expenditure with a large number of "0" values. According to the model, the medical expenditure of micro-individuals is determined by the probability model of medical treatment (the probit model is usually used to estimate) and the medical expenditure level model (the log formalized least square method, LOLS), and the two models are independent of each other, that is, the level of individual medical expenditure has nothing to do with whether they choose medical treatment or not.

Secondly, the Heckman sample selection model is mainly used to solve the problem that the authenticity and reliability of samples collected are reduced because the medical expenditures of middle-aged and elderly individuals are not incurred due to self-selection. The model consists of two parts: the selection equation, which mainly estimates whether an individual chooses to seek medical care (as shown in Equation (1)), and the expenditure equation, which is a regression estimate of the actual medical expenditure (as shown in Equation (2)).

$$P_i = \begin{cases} 1, & x_i\beta_1 + \varepsilon_{1i} > 0 \\ 0, & x_i\beta_1 + \varepsilon_{1i} \leq 0 \end{cases} \quad (1)$$

$$\log(y_i|p_i = 1) = x_i\beta_2 + \varepsilon_{2i} \quad (2)$$

When P_i takes is "0", it represents medical expenditure without medical treatment, while when P_i is "1", it represents medical expenditure with medical treatment.

Moreover, in order to deeply analyze the poverty reduction effect of medical insurance on middle-aged and elderly families, we use the Generalized Linear Model to carry out empirical research from two aspects: the absolute index (total medical expenditure) and the relative index (family medical financial burden). STATA 16 is used for all data processing in this paper.

2.4. Data Source

The research data of our paper comes from the 2018 tracking data released by the China Health and Retirement Longitudinal Survey (CHARLS) research group. CHARLS is a large-scale interdisciplinary research project hosted by the National Development Research Institute of Peking University. It collects high-quality micro-data of families and individuals of middle-aged and elderly people aged 45 and above in China over the years, covering more than 10,000 households in 150 counties and 450 villages in 28 provinces, to help scholars carry out interdisciplinary research on population aging and health issues. According to the public information of the research group, the updated tracking data will be released in 2023. By the end of 2022, the academic community will have produced more than 4000 academic achievements using the free and open database of the research group. A total of 3599 valid samples were screened out in this study.

3. Results

This paper uses the absolute index (total medical expenditure) and relative index (family medical financial burden, namely the proportion of medical expenditure in per capita annual income of the family) as the evaluation carriers. Among them, the relative index is at the core of discussing the poverty reduction effect.

3.1. Statistical Descriptive Analysis

Table 1 shows the descriptive statistics of the sample.

Table 1. Sample descriptive statistics.

Variable	Sample Size	Mean	Variance	Minimum	Maximum
Total medical expenditure	3599	7659.466	29,783.462	0	1,402,800
Family medical financial burden	3599	2.084	16.119	0	600
Number of chronic diseases	3599	1.121	1.258	0	9
Age	3599	63.807	9.972	45	95
Access to medical resources	3599	30.696	145.117	0	6000
Total annual household income	3599	32,292.177	75,975.197	2	1,930,000

As can be seen from Table 1, the self-rated health status of the mean is 0.597, which shows that most of the elderly's subjective health status is poor; objective health also has the same conclusion, chronic illness conditions in older adults indicate an average of 1.121 kinds of chronic diseases. Thus, the necessity for "healthy aging" in China is urgent. The average medical expenditure of the middle-aged and elderly is CNY 7659.466, which may be affected by special circumstances, and the average total medical expenditure is relatively high. The mean value of medical insurance participation is 0.815, indicating that the vast majority of those sampled participate in some kind of medical insurance at present, which is also consistent with the medical insurance participation situation published in China's current macro data. Sample description results in other explanatory variables show that the average age of the respondents is 63.807 years old, and most of them are rural residents with little education above primary school. The majority of those sampled are married, and the average annual household income is CNY 32,292.177. Most middle-aged and elderly people have no barriers to daily activities and they engage in moderate to high-intensity physical activity every week.

3.2. Absolute Index: Total Medical Expenditure

The empirical results are shown in Table 2.

Table 2. The substitution effect of medical insurance on total medical expenditure.

Variable	Two-Part Model		Heckman Sample Selection Model	
	Probability Model of Medical Treatment	Medical Expenditure Level Model	The Selection Equation	The Expenditure Equation
Medical insurance (uninsured as control group)	0.246	−0.259 **	0.168	−0.290 ***
	(0.184)	(0.101)	(0.177)	(0.103)
Male (female as control group)	−0.219	0.360 ***	−0.285 **	0.379 ***
	(0.142)	(0.0719)	(0.121)	(0.0732)
Age	−0.012	0.0258 ***	−0.018 **	0.027 ***
	(0.007)	(0.004)	(0.008)	(0.004)
Education level (no education as control group)				
Primary and below	0.240	−0.106	0.0778	−0.140
	(0.152)	(0.085)	(0.148)	(0.087)
Above primary school, secondary school, and below	0.505 **	0.086	0.125	0.0281
	(0.220)	(0.104)	(0.224)	(0.106)
Junior college or above	−0.052	−0.406	0.073	−0.374
	(0.381)	(0.275)	(0.301)	(0.278)
Married (single as control group)	0.253 *	0.204 **	0.130	0.165 *
	(0.152)	(0.094)	(0.131)	(0.095)
Access to medical resources	0.006	0.002 ***	0.011***	0.002 ***
	(0.004)	(0.000)	(0.004)	(0.000)
Log (total annual household income)	0.055	0.007	0.058	0.000
	(0.045)	(0.023)	(0.042)	(0.024)
Weekly physical activity (no exercise as control group)				
Low intensity	−0.183	−0.269 **	0.0435	−0.244 **
	(0.242)	(0.114)	(0.224)	(0.116)
Moderate intensity	−0.376	−0.462 ***	−0.146	−0.416 ***
	(0.247)	(0.117)	(0.227)	(0.119)
High intensity	−0.285	−0.737 ***	−0.088	−0.699 ***
	(0.258)	(0.121)	(0.237)	(0.123)
Self-rated health status (poor as control group)				
Fair	−0.017	−0.376 ***	−0.084	−0.375 ***
	(0.141)	(0.071)	(0.122)	(0.073)
Good	−0.279	−0.583 ***	−0.079	−0.539 ***
	(0.195)	(0.119)	(0.164)	(0.121)
Number of chronic diseases	0.088	0.134 ***	0.087	0.125 ***
	(0.060)	(0.027)	(0.054)	(0.027)
Constant	2.223 ***	6.237 ***	2.518 ***	6.306 ***
	(0.812)	(0.426)	(0.839)	(0.435)
Sample size	3599	3599	3599	3599

Note: * $p < 0.1$, ** $p < 0.05$, *** $p < 0.01$. Standard errors are in parentheses.

First of all, after controlling other variables, the impact of medical insurance on the medical expenditure of middle-aged and elderly people is mainly reflected in the expenditure model, while the probability of seeing a doctor selection equation shows that the influence coefficient of participation in medical insurance on the probability of medical treatment of the elderly is positive, but this result is not significant. The results of the expenditure equation show that the total medical expenditure of middle-aged and old people who have participated in medical insurance is significantly lower than that of middle-aged and old people who have not participated in medical insurance. The two-part model shows that participation in medical insurance will reduce the total medical expenditure by 25.9% at a significance level of 5%. The Heckman sample selection model shows a 29.0% reduction in total health spending, and the results are significant at the 1% level.

Secondly, there are other influencing factors. The medical expenditure level of middle-aged and elderly male groups is higher than that of female groups. The two-part model shows that the total medical expenditure of the male group is 36.0% higher than that of the female group, and the medical expenditure of males in the sample selection model is 37.9% higher than that of females. For each additional year of age, the total health spending increases by about 3%. In addition, there is no significant association between total health expenditure and educational level. Moderate exercise is beneficial in reducing the total medical expenditure of middle-aged and elderly people. Compared with the inactive middle-aged and elderly people, the medical expenditure of those who participate in moderate-intensity physical activity per week is reduced by more than 40%, and the medical expenditure of those who participate in high-intensity physical activity is reduced by 70% at a significance level of 1%.

In addition, medical expenditure and self-rated health status show a coincident change relationship. The higher the self-rated health, the lower the medical expenditure. People with average self-rated health spend about 37% less than those with poor self-rated health, and those with good self-rated health spend more than 50% less than those with poor self-rated health, which is significant at the 1% level. For each additional chronic illness, the two models show a 13.4% increase in total medical expenditure, and the Heckman sample selection model shows a 12.5% increase in total medical expenditure.

Therefore, the empirical results of the two-part model are basically consistent with the Heckman sample selection model, indicating that the empirical results are robust.

3.3. Relative Index: Family Medical Financial Burden

This section uses the relative index of the proportion of medical expenditure in the annual per capita income of families and evaluates the negative effect of medical insurance on the medical economic pressure of middle-aged and elderly families based on the characteristics of the index data combined with the generalized linear model. The regression results are shown in Table 3.

First of all, taking the group not participating in medical insurance as the control group, participating in medical insurance helps the middle-aged and elderly families reduce their medical financial burden by 3.47%, which is significant at the 5% significance level. Participation in medical insurance is beneficial in relieving the medical and economic pressure on middle-aged and elderly families.

Secondly, there are other influencing factors. The medical and financial pressure on middle-aged and elderly men is 4.17% higher than that of women ($p = 0.000$). With the increase in age, the medical financial burden of middle-aged and elderly families increases by 0.11%. The older the family is, the higher the medical expenditure is, and the heavier the medical financial burden is on the family. The coefficient of influence of the accessibility of medical resources on a family's medical financial burden is close to zero. The increase in family annual income is beneficial to reducing the medical financial burden of middle-aged and elderly families. In addition, the intensity of weekly physical activity has an impact on the family's medical financial burden. For example, participation in low-, moderate-, and high-intensity weekly physical activity is associated with a reduction of 3.96% ($p = 0.016$), 4.97% ($p = 0.003$), and 9.72% ($p = 0.000$) in family medical financial burden, respectively, compared with no physical activity.

Table 3. Research on the negative effect of medical insurance on the family medical financial burden.

Variable	Family Medical Financial Burden	Variable	Family Medical Financial Burden
Medical insurance (uninsured as control group)	−0.0347 ** (0.0145)	Married (single as control group)	−0.0002 (0.0135)
Male (female as control group)	0.0417 *** (0.0103)	Access to medical resources	0.0002 *** (0.0000)
Age	0.0011 * (0.0006)	Log (Total annual household income)	−0.1108 *** (0.0034)
Education level (no education as control group)		Weekly physical activity (No exercise control group)	
Primary and below	−0.0108 (0.0123)	Low intensity	−0.0396 ** (0.0164)
Above primary school, secondary school, and below	0.0034 (0.0149)	Moderate intensity	−0.0497 *** (0.0168)
Junior college or above	−0.0453 (0.0395)	High intensity	−0.0972 *** (0.0174)
Self-rated health status (poor as control group)		Number of chronic diseases	0.0131 *** (0.0038)
Fair	−0.0336 *** (0.0102)	Constant	1.9297 *** (0.0614)
Good	−0.0581 *** (0.0171)		

Note: * $p < 0.1$, ** $p < 0.05$, *** $p < 0.01$. Standard errors are in parentheses.

Third, the better the health status of the middle-aged and elderly, the lower the medical financial burden of their families. For each additional chronic disease, the financial burden of family health care increases by 1.31% (at the 1% significance level). The family medical financial burden of the middle-aged and old people with average self-rated health status is 3.36% lower than that of the middle-aged and old people with poor self-rated health status, and the family medical financial burden of the middle-aged and old people with poor self-rated health status is 5.81% lower.

3.4. Heterogeneity Analysis: Gender and Age

To test the heterogeneity of the impact of medical insurance proposed in some of the existing research results, this paper adopts the sub-sample regression method to conduct a classification regression according to the gender and age of the samples and to explore the group differences in the impact of medical insurance. The results are shown in Table 4.

Table 4. Heterogeneity analysis (gender differences and age differences).

		Observations	Total Medical Expenditure		Family Medical Financial Burden
			Probit	LOLS	
Gender differences	Female	2109	0.307 −0.271	−0.240 * −0.142	−0.029 −0.022
	Male	1490	0.194 −0.261	−0.261 * −0.145	−0.033 * −0.018
Age differences	Aged 45–59	1289	0.047 −0.464	0.009 0.182	0.002 0.031
	Aged 60 and above	2310	0.398 * −0.217	−0.374 *** −0.123	−0.047 *** −0.016

Note: * $p < 0.1$, *** $p < 0.01$. Standard errors are in parentheses.

First, gender differences are examined. Participation in medical insurance reduces the total medical expenditure of middle-aged and elderly females by 24.0% and that of middle-aged and elderly males by 26.1%, at a significance level of 10%, compared with the group that has not participated in medical insurance. This gender difference is also reflected in the impact on family medical burden. Participation in medical insurance reduces the family medical financial burden of a middle-aged and elderly male by 3.3%, this result is significant at the level of 10%, but the effect on the family medical financial burden of a middle-aged and elderly female is not significant. Therefore, the negative effect of medical insurance on the total medical expenditure of middle-aged and elderly males is slightly stronger than that of middle-aged and elderly females, and the negative effect on the family medical financial burden of middle-aged and elderly males is also stronger than that of females.

Second, the influence of age differences is explored. Participation in medical insurance has no significant effect on the 45–59 age group, but it can promote their utilization of health services for the elderly group aged 60 and above. It reduces their medical expenditure by 37.4% and their family medical economic burden by 4.7% at the significance level of 1%. This shows that the effect of medical insurance is more significant for the elderly group over 60 years.

4. Discussion

A high medical financial burden constitutes an important reason for some families to return to poverty, therefore, medical insurance plays an important role in preventing families from returning to poverty. This paper selected the middle-aged and elderly with a high demand for health services as the research object and the microdata of the latest CHARLS as the data source. Moreover, the poverty reduction effect of medical insurance on middle-aged and elderly families from the perspectives of the absolute index (total medical expenditure) and relative index (proportion of medical expenditure in per capita annual income) were discussed; some meaningful arguments were found.

First, there is a substitution effect between medical insurance and total medical expenditure. Similar to the research by Zang and Zhang (2019) [4] and Liu (2015) [9], medical insurance was found to be beneficial in significantly reducing the total medical expenditure of middle-aged and elderly people. The total medical expenditures of people with medical insurance were significantly lower than those of people who did not participate in medical insurance. In addition, the two-part model showed that participation in medical insurance reduced the total medical expenditure by 25.9% at a significance level of 5%. The Heckman sample selection model showed that participation in medical insurance resulted in a 29.0% reduction in total medical expenditure at a significance level of 1%. Two models were selected at the same time to better avoid the problem of sample endogeneity, and the empirical results obtained by the two empirical models were the same, indicating that the empirical results are relatively robust.

Second, medical insurance had a negative effect on middle-aged and elderly families. Medical insurance reduced the medical burden of middle-aged and elderly families. Compared with people who did not participate in medical insurance, participating in medical insurance helped them to reduce 2.36% of the medical financial burden at a 10% significance level, indicating that medical insurance may be beneficial for people by reducing medical expenditure by reducing precautionary savings. Although there are some differences in specific data, this further confirms the arguments of Ding and You (2019) [12] and Zhu and Shi (2016) [13].

Thirdly, the poverty reduction effect of medical insurance on middle-aged and elderly families had heterogeneity in gender and age. Compared with females, the negative effect of medical insurance was more significant for males. Participation in medical insurance reduced the total medical expenditure of middle-aged and elderly males more than that of middle-aged and elderly females. Medical insurance reduced the family medical burden of middle-aged and elderly males by 3.3% at a significance level of 10%, while the effect on the family medical burden of middle-aged and elderly females was not obvious.

Finally, appropriate participation in sports was beneficial for reducing the pressure of medical expenditures for the middle-aged and elderly. Compared with the middle-aged and elderly people who did not exercise, the total medical expenditure and family medical financial pressure of the middle-aged and elderly people who did exercise moderately every week was lower. In addition, taking part in low-intensity physical activity every week reduced the family's medical financial burden by 4.06% ($p = 0.004$), taking part in moderate-intensity physical activity every week reduced it by 6.03% ($p = 0.000$), and participation in high-intensity physical activity every week reduced it by 9.54% ($p = 0.000$). Therefore, our conclusion is the same as Ren et al. (2014) [22]: participation in physical activity significantly reduced the pressure of medical expenditure on middle-aged and elderly people by reducing their probability of illness.

However, there are inevitably some study limitations. For example, a longitudinal comparative study on the historical data of CHARLS (2008, 2011, 2015, and 2018) was not conducted; perhaps the longitudinal research results of the multi-year data are more accurate. In addition, our research data is taken from the 2018 data, before the outbreak of COVID-19 which has had a huge impact on China's national economy and households over the past three years and may also cause some deviation from our research conclusions.

Nevertheless, our research still brings some policy implications. First, the government should further expand medical insurance coverage to ease financial burden and promote equal access to health. For example, the government should strengthen the publicity of the important role of medical insurance, especially for middle-aged and elderly individuals with poor health, and there should be a large demand for medical services to participate more in medical insurance so that they can enjoy the welfare policies of medical insurance, improve the overall health level of the people, and relieve the pressure of rising medical expenses. Secondly, the government should give more protection to vulnerable groups, such as the elderly and low-income families, and improve the fairness and effectiveness of the medical insurance system. The effect of medical insurance on the medical expenditure of middle-aged and elderly families is more significant than in urban and high-income groups. Therefore, the marginal utility of medical insurance for the middle-aged and elderly and low-income groups is higher. From the perspective of improving the fairness and efficiency of the system, medical insurance should be strengthened in the protection of vulnerable insured groups by expanding the coverage of low-income groups, reducing the proportion of self-payment and other measures, and providing more welfare policies to middle-aged and elderly people and low-income groups. Finally, the government should improve the supporting mechanism of medical insurance and the medical security system. Although medical insurance reduces the medical burden of the insured object, the effect is limited. With the rapid increase in the care and medical needs of the disabled elderly, it is urgent to introduce corresponding countermeasures, such as the promotion of long-term care insurance policies, to effectively disperse the pressure faced by medical insurance.

5. Conclusions

Our research results further verify that medical insurance can significantly reduce the total medical expenditure of middle-aged and elderly people, thus reducing the medical burden of middle-aged and elderly families. That is, medical insurance has a poverty reduction effect on middle-aged and elderly families, and there is heterogeneity in gender and age. Accordingly, we propose to further expand the scope of medical insurance to provide more protection for the elderly and low-income families, as well as other vulnerable groups, and improve the fairness and effectiveness of the medical insurance system. However, the pressure of government financial expenditure (especially under the impact of continuous COVID-19), the existence of a moral hazard, and other factors have reduced the effectiveness of medical insurance. The long-term care insurance system, which is relatively mature in Germany, Japan, and other developed countries but has only begun to pilot in China in 2016, can play a certain auxiliary role.

Future academic research can be further expanded in the following aspects: first, integrate the latest CHARLS data with previous data to explore the changing process of the poverty reduction effect of medical insurance on middle-aged and elderly families. Second, focus on adverse selection and moral hazard in medical insurance and evaluate the impact of adverse selection and moral hazard on the release effect and negative effect of medical insurance demand. Third, evaluate the tacit degree and actual effectiveness of various medical insurance divisions and cooperations, combined with other medical insurance systems in China, and explore the overall improvement plan of the current medical insurance system in China, including further improvement of the auxiliary role of the long-term nursing insurance system.

Author Contributions: Methodology, L.C.; Data analysis, L.C.; Writing the first draft, X.X.; Editing and review, L.C.; Project administration, X.X. All authors have read and agreed to the published version of the manuscript.

Funding: This paper is a phased achievement of The National Social Science Fund of China: Research on the blocking mechanism of the Borderline poor families returning to poverty due to illness, No: 20BJY057.

Institutional Review Board Statement: The data of this study came from the China Health and Retirement Longitudinal Survey (CHARLS), which Peking University sponsored. It was ethically reviewed by the Biomedical Ethics Committee, Peking University, Ethics Review, with Approval No. IRB00001052-11015. We also obtained confirmation that the need for ethical applications was waived by the CHARLS research team, since CHARLS is an open and accessible (publicly-available) database, and the authors only used the data for academic research.

Informed Consent Statement: Not applicable.

Data Availability Statement: Please refer to: http://charls.pku.edu.cn/index.html (accessed on 16 May 2021).

Acknowledgments: Thanks to The National School of Development and The Chinese Center for Social Science Surveys at Peking University for providing CHARLS data. We also thank Zhang Lu and Yang Haoran (postgraduate students), for their contributions to data collation and empirical study.

Conflicts of Interest: The authors declare no conflict of interest.

References

1. Xu, X.; Huang, X. Risk Characteristics of Catastrophic Health Expenditure in Multidimensional Borderline Poor Households in China. *Risk Manag. Healthc. Policy* **2023**, *16*, 15–29. [CrossRef] [PubMed]
2. Antwi, Y.A.; Moriya, A.S.; Simon, K.I. Access to health insurance and the use of inpatient medical care: Evidence from the Affordable Care Act young adult mandate. *J. Health Econ.* **2015**, *39*, 171–187. [CrossRef] [PubMed]
3. Si, W. Public health insurance and the labor market: Evidence from China's Urban Resident Basic Medical Insurance. *Health Econ.* **2021**, *30*, 403–431. [CrossRef] [PubMed]
4. Zang, X.; Zhang, Q. Health insurance and household consumption from the perspective of intergenerational support: An analysis based on generation overlapping Model. *J. Shandong Univ.* **2019**, *1*, 15–24. (In Chinese)
5. Jung, J.; Streeter, J.L. Does health insurance decrease health expenditure risk in developing countries? The case of China. *South. Econ. J.* **2015**, *82*, 361–384. [CrossRef]
6. Kang, H.A.; Barner, J.C. The relationship between out-of-pocket healthcare expenditures and insurance status among individuals with chronic obstructive pulmonary disease. *J. Pharm. Health Serv. Res.* **2017**, *8*, 107–113. [CrossRef]
7. Choi, J.W.; Park, E.C.; Lee, S.G.; Park, S.; Ryu, H.-G.; Kim, T.H. Does long-term care insurance reduce the burden of medical costs? A retrospective elderly cohort study. *Geriatr. Gerontol. Int.* **2018**, *18*, 1641–1646. [CrossRef]
8. Feng, J.; Wang, Z.; Yu, Y. Does long-term care insurance reduce hospital utilization and medical expenditures? Evidence from China. *Soc. Sci. Med.* **2020**, *258*, 113081. [CrossRef]
9. Liu, M.; Qiu, C. Performance evaluation of medical insurance on hospsitalization behavior and burden of elderly population: Based on The Chinese Health and pension Tracking Surve. *Insur. Res.* **2014**, *9*, 58–70. (In Chinese)
10. Meng, Y.; Zhang, X.; Han, J. The impact of medical insurance programmes on the health of the insured: Evidence from China. *Int. J. Health Plan. Manag.* **2020**, *35*, 718–734. [CrossRef]

11. Huang, X.; Wu, C. Research on the Crowding out effect of social medical insurance on preventive savings. *World Econ.* **2006**, *8*, 65–70. (In Chinese)
12. Ding, J.; You, L. Research on the impact of basic medical insurance on catastrophic health expenditure of the elderly. *Insur. Res.* **2019**, *12*, 98–107. (In Chinese)
13. Zhu, M.; Shi, X. Impact of medical insurance on catastrophic medical expenditure of Floating Population. *Chin. J. Popul. Sci.* **2016**, *6*, 47–57. (In Chinese)
14. Alkenbrack, S.; Lindelow, M. The Impact of Community-Based Health Insurance on Utilization and Out-of-Pocket Expenditures in Lao People's Democratic Republic. *Health Econ.* **2015**, *24*, 379–399. [CrossRef]
15. Jin, S.; Yu, J. The influence of medical insurance system on income distribution: A Case study of Shaanxi Province. *Chin. J. Popul. Sci.* **2017**, *3*, 116–125+128. (In Chinese)
16. Yu, D.; Wu, Y.; Zhao, X. The influence of social medical insurance on elderly's medical consumption and health: An evaluation of institutional Effect and analysis of its mechanism. *J. Financ. Econ.* **2018**, *34*, 149–160. (In Chinese)
17. Chen, Y.; Shi, J.; Zhuang, C.C. Income-dependent impacts of health insurance on medical expenditures: Theory and evidence from China. *China Econ. Rev.* **2019**, *53*, 290–310. [CrossRef]
18. Kwon, E.; Park, S.; McBride, T.D. Health Insurance and Poverty in Trajectories of Out-of-Pocket Expenditure among Low-Income Middle-Aged Adults. *Health Serv. Res.* **2018**, *53*, 4332–4352. [CrossRef]
19. Li, L.; Yu, Q. Research on the impact of the reform of payment mode of basic medical insurance on medical expenses in China. *Comp. Econ. Soc. Syst.* **2019**, *2*, 69–80. (In Chinese)
20. Wang, N.; Gao, W.; Ma, M.; Shan, L.; Fu, X.; Sun, T.; Xia, Q.; Tian, W.; Liu, L.; Yang, H.; et al. The medical insurance system's weakness to provide economic protection for vulnerable citizens in China: A five-year longitudinal study. *Arch. Gerontol. Geriatr.* **2021**, *92*, 104227. [CrossRef]
21. Yang, M. Demand for social health insurance: Evidence from the Chinese new rural cooperative medical scheme. *China Econ. Rev.* **2018**, *52*, 126–135. [CrossRef]
22. Ren, Y.; Kan, X.; Song, D. Adverse selection and moral hazard: A Review of the basic medical insurance market for the elderly. *J. Shanghai Univ. Financ. Econ.* **2014**, *16*, 54–63. (In Chinese)
23. Zhao, S.; Zhang, X.; Dai, W.; Ding, Y.-X.; Chen, J.-Y.; Fang, P.-Q. Effect of the catastrophic medical insurance on household catastrophic health expenditure: Evidence from China. *Gac. Sanit.* **2021**, *34*, 370–376. [CrossRef] [PubMed]
24. Cao, X.; Tan, X. Integration of medical insurance for urban and rural residents and health of middle-aged and elderly people in rural areas: An empirical study based on CHARLS data. *J. Agric. Technol. Econ.* **2022**, *12*, 56–70. (In Chinese)
25. Xu, X.; Gu, H. Impact of critical illness insurance on medical utilization and health of middle-aged and elderly residents: An empirical test based on CHARLS data. *Popul. Dev.* **2022**, *28*, 16–29. (In Chinese)

Disclaimer/Publisher's Note: The statements, opinions and data contained in all publications are solely those of the individual author(s) and contributor(s) and not of MDPI and/or the editor(s). MDPI and/or the editor(s) disclaim responsibility for any injury to people or property resulting from any ideas, methods, instructions or products referred to in the content.

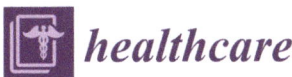

Article

Towards Cultural Adequacy of Experience-Based Design: A Qualitative Evaluation of Community-Integrated Intermediary Care to Enhance the Family-Based Long-Term Care for Thai Older Adults

Thin Nyein Nyein Aung [1,2], Thaworn Lorga [3], Saiyud Moolphate [4], Yuka Koyanagi [5], Chaisiri Angkurawaranon [1,2], Siripen Supakankunti [6], Motoyuki Yuasa [7,8] and Myo Nyein Aung [4,7,8,9,*]

1. Department of Family Medicine, Faculty of Medicine, Chiang Mai University, Chiang Mai 50200, Thailand; drthinnyeinaung@gmail.com (T.N.N.A.); chaisiri.a@cmu.ac.th (C.A.)
2. Global Health and Chronic Conditions Research Group, Chiang Mai University, Chiang Mai 50200, Thailand
3. Faculty of Nursing, Chiang Mai Rajabhat University, Mae Hong Son Campus, Mae Hong Son 58000, Thailand; thaworn.lorga@gmail.com
4. Department of Public Health, Faculty of Science and Technology, Chiang Mai Rajabhat University, Chiang Mai 50300, Thailand; saiyudmoolphate@gmail.com
5. Department of Judo Therapy, Faculty of Medical and Health Sciences, Tokyo Ariake University of Medical and Health Sciences, Tokyo 135-0063, Japan; koyanagiy@tau.ac.jp
6. Centre of Excellence for Health Economics, Faculty of Economics, Chulalongkorn University, Bangkok 10330, Thailand; siripen.s@chula.ac.th
7. Department of Global Health Research, Graduate School of Medicine, Juntendo University, Tokyo 113-8421, Japan; moyuasa@juntendo.ac.jp
8. Faculty of International Liberal Arts, Juntendo University, Tokyo 113-8421, Japan
9. Advanced Research Institute for Health Sciences, Juntendo University, Tokyo 113-8421, Japan
* Correspondence: myo@juntendo.ac.jp

Abstract: In this qualitative study, we provided an in-depth understanding of how Community-Integrated Intermediary Care (CIIC), a new service model for family-based long-term care (LTC), was perceived by its users. The CIIC, established in Chiang Mai, Northern Thailand, consisted of three main interventions: (1) A temporary respite care center, (2) A family centered care capacity building; (3) Functional training delivered as community group exercise and home exercise to improve healthy ageing for independent older adults. Ten pairs of dependent Thai older adults, their primary family caregivers, and ten village health volunteers were recruited using the purposive sampling method. Data were collected via semistructured in-depth interviews. A thematic descriptive qualitative analysis was used for data analysis. The findings revealed that CIIC helped reduce the burden of family caregivers by providing respite, relief, and care coordination. The experiences of the CIIC users indicated possibilities for service redesign, development, and delivery strategies to better meet the LTC needs of older adults and family caregivers. Following the local stakeholders' commitment and local community health volunteers' network, a well-integrated formal and informal care CIIC model can be implied as an effective and sustainable ageing care service model in Thailand and other Asian countries in the future.

Keywords: ageing; caregiving; Community-Integrated Intermediary Care (CIIC); older adult; Thailand

1. Introduction

Population ageing is increasing worldwide [1,2] and Thailand is expected to step into the super-aged society as the percentage of Thailand's total population aged over 60 years old is estimated to reach 28% by 2031 [3]. The sustainability of the traditional family-based long-term care model, currently practiced in Thailand and other Asian countries, has been challenged by the rapidly ageing population, increasing skipped generations where grandparents are left at home with their grandchildren to take care of each other reciprocally, and increasing direct and indirect cost from informal caregiving by the family members [4–7]. To address these challenges in sustainability through human resources and technical needs, a randomized controlled trial, Community Integrated Intermediary Care (TCTR20190412004; Thailand (CIIC project)) was implemented in Chiang Mai where 18.2% of the total population comprised older adults [8].

The CIIC center was established in February 2020 on a campus of the Mae Hia Municipality, Chiang Mai, Northern Thailand. This new service model, serving as an intermediary care center, was situated and integrated within the local community. The intermediary care concept would link families and communities to formal local older adult care services and funding within each municipality. The CIIC center, an intervention component of the research trial, was a result of the coordinated efforts between Japanese and Thai academics, local government, and health care providers [9,10]. The Japanese team offered technical and financial support, while the Thai team allowed the use of physical spaces and established the needed mechanisms for the operation of the CIIC center. The efforts were aimed at responding to the challenges imposed by the lack of innovative and alternative long-term care (LTC) services amidst an increasing number of Thai older persons and families with complex LTC needs. The CIIC project was set out to provide the following services: screening and assessment of family caregiver burden and LTC capacity, care capacity building for family caregivers, care prevention exercise program for independent older persons, and respite care service for families having difficulties with caregiving for dependent older adults with functional limitations, measured by using Barthel's activities of daily living (ADL). The primary outcome was to reduce family caregivers' burden. The secondary outcomes included improvements in ADL, depression, and quality of life of older adult participants.

1.1. Physical Spaces of the CIIC

The center was set up in a building adjacent to the main building of the Mae Hia Municipality. The CIIC room measured 6×4 m^2 and was accessible via a main entrance door and an exit door at the rear. It was furnished with four beds, a dining table, and two recliners. Optimal room temperature was maintained by two air conditioners and two fans. Mobile curtains were provided to maintain privacy when needed. A toilet specifically designed for people with mobility impairments was installed.

1.2. The COVID-19 Pandemic and the Implementation of the CIIC Project

Despite a very solid implementation plan, the CIIC project could not be fully implemented due to the COVID-19 pandemic in Thailand. With the emergency declaration on 26 March 2020 [11], and COVID-19 pandemic containment measures, we stopped the activity from March until the end of June 2020. For safety concerns of the people and all parties involved in the implementation, the community-based care prevention group exercise activities were replaced by a home exercise program. A home exercise DVD, poster, and dairy calendar were provided by the CIIC project. Home visits and technical training to enhance the care capacity of family caregivers in need were also interrupted by social distancing measures during the COVID-19 pandemic. However, the research team continued to monitor the burdened family caregivers and provided tailor-made technical guidance via an online platform. The implementation was reassessed from time to time due to the COVID-19 situation. Unfortunately, as the pandemic remained serious and unpredictable, the CIIC center's ability to accept dependent older adults with burdened family caregivers was put on hold indefinitely for safety reasons and to comply with the government measures to curb infection rates. To plan for reimplementation and to ensure the best fit of the CIIC services postpandemic, we conducted a qualitative study to gauge unique experiences of older adults, families, and service providers. Taking the experience-based design (EBD) approach [12–14], we aimed to identify the implications for improving or revising the originally planned CIIC services. The EBD approach is a method of capturing experiences and designing better service encounters leading to satisfaction and wellbeing for those using and delivering health and social services. Despite CIIC not being implemented fully, we aimed to explore the understanding of older adults, families, and stakeholders' views on CIIC as it is necessary to estimate the extent of their acceptability of CIIC and to identify other potential benefits of the CIIC center apart from those highlighted in the proposal.

2. Materials and Methods

2.1. Ethics, Study Design, and Participants

This study was conducted following the Declaration of Helsinki [15]. The World Health Organization Ethical Review Committee (WHO/ERC ID; ERC.0003064, dated 7 March 2019) and Ethical Review Committee for Research in Human Subjects, Boromarajonani College of Nursing Nakhon Lampang, Praboromarajchanok under the Institute for Health Workforce Development, Ministry of Public Health, Thailand (approval number E 2562/005, dated 4 March 2019) approved the ethics of the study. It has been registered at the Thailand Clinical Trial Registry, trial registration number TCTR20190412004. We conducted face-to-face in-depth interviews, using semistructured questionnaires with 10 pairs of Thai older adults and their primary family caregivers and 10 village health volunteers (VHVs) via door-to-door home visits. Older adults have been defined as participants aged 60 years completed and above. The primary family caregiver is defined as the family member who spends the most time providing unpaid care to the dependent care recipients and who is perceived by themselves and others as the principal person responsible for caring for older adults. Village health volunteers, the heart of primary healthcare works, have been playing a key role as community health workers in the primary healthcare system in Thailand for many decades [16]. Based on the Thai cultural ideals of volunteerism and helping each other, VHVs are key community personnel in the delivery of care for older adults with chronic diseases [17]. By using the purposive sampling method, potential participants were approached and asked by a community volunteer if they were interested in participating in the interview. Those who expressed their interest were notified of the nature of their participation in the study and they were advised that their participation in the study would not have any impact on their current or future provision of healthcare. All the participants that were approached agreed to participate in the project and consented to their participation. Each participant was interviewed once at their home by a trained qualitative researcher. To improve quality assurance and to avoid investigator bias, qualitative inquiry and analysis were led by an external expert. The families and older adults were shown a set of pictures of the CIIC center, which was easily accessible and located within their local community. Afterward, we asked them to reflect on specific issues such as how they liked the ideas of CIIC, what they expected from the CIIC center, their contributions to the services, and their preferences for the services and the physical structure of the room. The caregiver interview was guided by a series of open-ended requests and questions: (1) Please tell me of your experience (in the past and at the present) with caregiving of the older person; (2) What are the negative and positive sides of your caregiving? (optional); (3) Please tell me of your experience with CIIC and its utilization; (4) What should we do to improve your caregiving experience? (5) What should we do to make CIIC work for you? The older adult participant was simply asked "In what regards do you think the CIIC has helped you and your family?" The VHVs were asked about their roles in CIIC, the roles of CIIC in long-term care, and the improvements needed. Following their responses to these guided questions, additional in-depth questions were used to elicit their responses in detail.

2.2. Data Analysis

In-depth interview transcripts were audio-recorded and transcribed into English. Participants were deidentified and assigned study-specific codes to exclude their names and any other identifying details in any study data electronic file to secure the confidentiality of participation. Data analysis was carried out via manual qualitative analysis using thematic charts [18–21]. Trustworthiness of qualitative analysis was ensured according to the four criteria identified by Lincoln and Guba [22]: credibility (e.g., frequent debriefing sessions among researchers); transferability (e.g., comparison with previous literature); and dependability and confirmability (e.g., using replicable methods, detailed description of the study protocol). Thematic descriptive qualitative analysis of the data took the following steps. For each interview transcript, two researchers read through the whole transcript to capture the holistic picture of the participant's experience. These two analysts then identified the smallest units of data together and assigned them a meaningful code (called open coding). The open codings with similar meanings were then grouped into subthemes. Lastly, subthemes were grouped into a theme. The two analysts discussed subthemes and themes to maximize the best fit between the themes and subthemes and their respective coding of the participant's quotes. The analysts then checked whether the themes and subthemes reflected the participants' experiences. These themes and subthemes were modified via subsequent analyses. As a result, there were four themes and eleven subthemes to identify the additional features of CIIC to meet the needs of Thai older adults, their families, and other stakeholders for the future implementation of CIIC.

3. Results

The study participants included bedridden older adults (Barthel's ADL score 0–4), with the most common underlying condition of stroke, followed by cancer, dementia, and hip fracture. Primary family caregivers are mostly constituted of spouses and children with a mean age of 55.27 ± 13.7 years. The VHVs were mostly middle-aged well-to-do persons with their own businesses, such as grocery shop owners, booksellers, food kiosk owners, florists, etc. Four themes were identified from interviews with family caregivers, Thai older adults, and volunteers. The themes are as follows: (1) Becoming a good caregiver; (2) Stretching to the limit; (3) Taking care of one's health; (4) The roles of CIIC in addressing gaps in care and strengthening care systems. A summary of the emergent themes, subthemes, and participants' quotes is described in Table 1.

Table 1. A summary of the emergent themes and participants' quotes in qualitative descriptive analysis.

	Themes Summary	Participants' Quotes
Theme 1	Becoming a good caregiver	
Subtheme 1	A responsibility to care: family caregivers began with being assigned a responsibility to care for dependent older adults regardless of their readiness or preparation to take on this duty of care.	"He is my husband. It's my responsibility to take care of him. It can't be the others." (FCG ID 1)
		"I am tired of caregiving, but I am happy as I must return for spending her life to take care of her children when we were young." (FCG ID 2)
		"It's a family responsibility. We can't deny it or expect others to do it for us." (FCG ID 8)
Subtheme 2	Mastering oneself as a caregiver: The process of caregiving mastering is not static. Rather, it is quite dynamic and dependent upon the changing needs of older adults as their illnesses change.	"Every day is a learning day for me. I learned about the disease that he got. I learned about his medications. I learned everything that I need to learn to look after him well. I practiced and learned many skills to help him with daily tasks. It's a lot easier now [than in the past] to help him through the day." (FCG ID 1)
		"You get better at it [caregiving task] the next time you do it. I felt it was challenging at the beginning, but I think I'm pretty good at it now." (FCG ID 4)

Table 1. Cont.

	Themes Summary	Participants' Quotes
Subtheme 3	Applying the knowledge and skills in caregiving: the acquired knowledge and caregiving skills are sometimes applied through a trial-and-error process.	"The doctors and nurses would give us a lot of advice and knowledge. But we need to make it fit with the care recipient. It's not always like what the doctors said to us." (FCG ID 4)
		"Our house is very small, and it is packed with our stuff. There are steps all over the place. Getting around in a wheelchair inside the house is almost impossible. We need to use tandem walking quite a lot to help her move around the house. We tied a rope around her waist to make tandem walking easier and safe [so she would not fall]." (FCG ID 3)
Subtheme 4	Knowing the care recipients: it is one of the critical aspects for the quality of care for older adults with long-term complex care needs.	"He was barely talking. So, we had to guess what made him look unhappy and restless. We had to try different things to help him. Many things didn't work. But finally, we would find something that worked for him. You need to know the older people. I think each person is unique. You must be a good observer and attentive to care for them well." (FCG ID 1)
		"When she frowns and moves her legs, I know there must be something wrong with her. I would check whether she wet or soil herself first as this is often the case when she behaves like this." (FCG ID 10)
Theme 2	Stretching to the limit	
Subtheme 1	Everything is centered around the care recipient: the needs of care recipients are prioritized over other needs.	"It's always about her. It [caring for her] is the priority. We must settle her care first before we do something else." (FCG ID 2)
		"Everyone asks about their patient but not so much about us [caregivers]. They would ask whether the care recipient progresses well or has any problems. I understand that we have very limited time during each consultation [at the hospital] so we need to focus on the care recipient." (FCG ID 3)
Subtheme 2	Meeting caregiving burdens and demands at all costs	"We would do everything to keep him well. Anything that we can afford even though it is hard. Physically, financially, and emotionally." (FCG ID 9)
		"My dad has been bedridden for about three years, and I used all my time and efforts to take care of him. It was very difficult for me to make proper positioning, transfer, and mobility before I got specific guidance from the CIIC team. Thank you and because of the improvement in caregiving skills, I can spare some time to take care of myself every day." (FCG ID 4)
		"I need to sacrifice a lot. I had to quit my job in the city to be her caregiver. Now I don't have a monthly salary. I opened a food kiosk at home so I can be with her and have some regular income." (FCG ID 3)
Subtheme 3	Impacts of caregiving on caregivers and family functioning	"I suddenly became jobless when both of my parents got bedridden as I am the only child to take care of them. I did not feel guilty about quitting my job, but I was exhausted from caregiving." (FCG ID 8)
		"I don't have time to myself. In fact, the whole family doesn't have time for us. We have no life outside our home. No more gatherings with friends. It can be tough sometimes." (FCG ID 9)

Table 1. *Cont.*

	Themes Summary	Participants' Quotes
		"There are ups and downs all the time. This was especially at the beginning of her illness. A lot was happening then. There were times when I felt that it was too much. I am coping much better now but I can expect a time when I feel low." (FCG ID 2)
		"We have to juggle the care tasks and other things. It's a constant planning and decision making." (FCG ID 7)
Theme 3	Taking care of one's health	
Subtheme 1	Healthy lifestyles applied and better health realized by caregivers	"Taking care of others has taught me a lot about the importance of having good health. If you don't want to go down that path [being bedridden], you must look after your health very well. I am careful about what I eat. I try to go for a walk whenever I have time." (FCG ID 5)
		"I could get advice from the CIIC team not only for specific caregiving skills such as bed bathing, occupied bed making, etc. but also nutrition advice on how to prepare a balanced diet for my mother". (FCG ID 2)
		"I have my blood pressure taken by the volunteer as often as I can. I weigh myself at least once a week, so I know what my body is like." (FCG ID 8)
		"One of the good things about being a caregiver is that I have better health. My muscles are much firmer now, and I feel a lot healthier because of following the healthy lifestyle." (FCG ID 10)
Theme 4	Roles of CIIC in addressing gaps in care and strengthening care systems	
Subtheme 1	Fragmentation in formal health and social services: having multiple health providers also contributed to fragmentation in care as there was no overall governing body responsible for the long-term care of older people.	"There were many hurdles that we had to go through to get things we wanted for the older adult. We [the family] had to navigate the [health and social] services by ourselves. The services were there but we needed to connect them. To do that, we had to communicate with different people again and again. You know, there are two separate systems that we must go through. It's not a smooth process at all." (FCG ID 3)
		"Information from different health providers can be inconsistent. It's up to us to decide which one is right for us. No one knows the whole picture of the care recipient. They seem to know parts of it, so it's hard to get everything done in one go." (FCG ID 4)
Subtheme 2	A dedicated and devoted volunteer is instrumental in care management	"Without the volunteer, our family would not be able to stand on our own feet now. She is so supportive. She is always there for us. She helps talk to the local government and visits us often. She is the one who cares enough to ask us how we are." (FCG ID 1)
		"She is the one who makes sure patients and families in need of support get help. She has a strong sense of community where everyone cares for everyone. She helps promote our foods in the community so that we can have a good sale and earn more money." (FCG ID 4)
		"I am proud of myself to be a health care volunteer to assist burdened families with dependent older adults. I assumed that this is our duty to take care of each other in the local community." (Volunteer ID 4)

Table 1. Cont.

	Themes Summary	Participants' Quotes
		"I am a retired person and I have plenty of free time to take care of my neighbors. I am happy to contribute some good things to my village." (Volunteer ID 1)
		"When I noticed that she locked her father in bed, I know it is not good care. I think it is our responsibility to help burdened families in our community." (Volunteer ID 6)
		"I am happy as I can do CIIC exercise and encourage my friends to do so." (Volunteer ID 8)
Subtheme 3	Acceptability of the CIIC: The proposed CIIC and its services are very well appreciated and accepted by families, older adults, and volunteers. The CIIC center is viewed as an alternative to respite care, not as a replacement for family care. Home-based care is still the best option for families and older adults.	"Thank you. I feel pity for my son for taking care of me all the time. I want him to take a break. I am pleased to hear that I can stay there for one week." (Older adult ID 4) "It is located within our village. I think I can stay happily there for a short time but not for a long time." (Older adult ID 5) "I don't want to stay there. I have decided to stay at home until my last breath. Please come to help my daughter who is tired of caregiving." (Older adult ID 8) "Is it expensive? I noticed she is using a lot of money for buying things for me including diapers and skin lotions. If it is free of charge care, I want to stay there for a while." (Older adult ID 9) "When I heard about the CIIC project where we can send our dependent care recipients for a short-term stay, I felt a big relief, even though I could not have a chance to use their respite care service because of the COVID-19 situation." (FCG ID 8)
		"I think free-of-charge care can be difficult to sustain long term. You better charge the rich family to use your CIIC center services." (FCG ID 3)
		"I like the idea of CIIC center as it is located within our village and my mother may not feel being away from home." (FCG ID 7)
		"I felt encouraged when I heard that I could send my mother to your care center temporarily. Thank you." (FCG ID 10)

Note: FCG = Primary Family Caregiver.

3.1. Theme 1: Becoming a Good Caregiver

Caregivers of older adults in need of LTC at home have gone through a recognizable pattern of caregiving experiences. It is important to note that, in most cases, only one family member was selected as the principal caregiver. The sole principal caregiver had to shoulder the caregiving responsibility and tasks throughout their developmental career as a caregiver. Family caregivers began with being assigned a responsibility to care for dependent older adults regardless of their readiness or preparation to take on this duty of care. They may or may not be adequately prepared by a hospital or healthcare facility. As a result of the healthcare providers' lack of knowledge of the whole picture of the situations and contexts in which care was taking place, most of these existing services could not meet the information and instrumental needs of the care recipients and their families. Therefore, informational, educational, and training services tended to be one-size-fits-all services. It was very common for family caregivers to seek additional information and knowledge to provide proper care to their dependent older adults. This often resulted in caregivers receiving incomplete, untailored (too general), and conflicting information which made it difficult for them to use the knowledge in managing care. Apart from the information, caregivers also had to acquire the skills required to work with older adults. These skills included skills related to medical procedures, moving, or transferring the care recipients, waste management, nutrition and hydration management, hygiene care, self-care assistance, and communication. The process of mastering caregiving is not static. It is rather a dynamic process as it is dependent upon the changing needs of older adults as their illnesses change. The vast knowledge and skills the family caregivers have received either through health service providers or self-inquiries are put into play. The acquired knowledge and skills were sometimes applied through a trial-and-error process. This process may take weeks or months before the caregivers can figure out what works best for the patient, for them, and their family. Knowing the care recipient was one of the critical aspects for the quality of care for older adults with complex LTC needs. As the caregivers became more involved and engaged with their caregiving, they observed the care recipients and learned about their behaviors, problems, and needs. They also learned what works and what does not. Knowing the care recipients not only helped increase the quality of care but also reduced caregivers' frustration because of trial and error. It also improved the caregivers' confidence and morale as they have achieved the desired outcomes of care.

3.2. Theme 2: Stretching to the Limit

To meet the needs of older adults, family caregivers must stretch their limits. The situation was particularly stressful for families living with very limited incomes, irregular jobs and earnings, and a limited number of capable caregivers. This also applied to caregivers having ill health and chronic conditions which need to be managed. Everything was centered around the care recipient and their needs were prioritized over other needs of the caregivers. Caregivers were trying their best to put the needs of their care recipients ahead of theirs. Healthcare providers also focused solely on the needs of the dependent older adults without extending specific considerations to the needs of caregivers or families. Healthcare assessments were purely directed at the care recipients, leaving very limited room for discussions about the caregivers' family situations and wellbeing. Having to stretch their limits can negatively impact the family's functionality, wellbeing, and the quality of care provided to their care recipients. Negative impacts of caregiving on different aspects of their life were noted, one of which was loss of a job due to voluntary job resignation to become a caregiver. In addition, others experienced a loss of economic productivity as they had to juggle between jobs and caregiving tasks. They also experienced muscle pains and aches, emotional stresses, social isolation, and lack of sleep.

3.3. Theme 3: Taking Care of One's Health: Healthy Lifestyles Applied and Better Health Realized by the Caregivers

Despite evidence of negative experiences of caregivers about caregiving, they also reported positive aspects of caregiving. Being a caregiver for a certain period made the caregiver and the family health conscious. The caregivers learned about healthy lifestyle choices, applied what they learned by themselves, and realized the benefits of adopting healthy lifestyles. Understanding healthy foods and diets was the most common benefit highlighted by the primary family caregivers.

3.4. Theme 4: Roles of CIIC in Addressing Gaps in Care and Strengthening Care Systems

Caregivers experienced fragmentation in existing health services, especially during the early stages of caregiving. The early stages of caregiving often involved decision-making on health services, settlements of jobs and caregiving demands, and caregiving arrangements. This stage featured high emotional stress among caregivers due to the abrupt changes and crises in the family. Caregivers found it difficult to sort out all the information in a way that eased their decisions. Having multiple healthcare providers also contributed to the fragmentation of care as there was no overall governing body responsible for the LTC of older adults. There were also no specific focal point service providers who could navigate the caregivers into the system or liaise the services across different care systems. A stark fragmentation was found between health and social service systems. Bridging the two systems needed to be fulfilled by the families themselves. This often-caused unnecessary stress on the caregivers and delayed access to the required services and help. In the absence of comprehensive social services, caused by a lack of an effective coordination system between health and social care, dedicated and devoted volunteers became critical in liaising between the two systems. A dedicated and devoted volunteer is valuable and instrumental to care management. Volunteers helped communicate with the local government about the unmet needs of the care recipient older adults and caregiving families, raised community awareness about the families in need of support, conducted regular visits to their houses and assessed the ongoing problems and needs, connected families to existing resources within and outside the community, assisted the families to the extent of job and income generation, and spoke for the families. Their dedicated efforts have seen older adults receive the needed services from the local government such as home modifications and financial assistance. The proposed CIIC and its services were very well appreciated and accepted by families, older adults, and volunteers. The CIIC center was viewed as an alternative to respite care, not a replacement for family care. Home-based care is still the best option for families and older adults as the care recipients and caregivers prefer to be cared for in their own homes. Being in their own home is associated with having control of what they do, conveniently accessing needed items, and being less stressed due to the familiar surroundings and people at home. CIIC respite service is the perfect option when the family cannot juggle between routines and caregiving tasks. Respite care has a short-term stay nature, not a long-term continuous stay, and it is free of charge. Voluntary donations to the center should be considered an alternative to fixed-cost copayment. Proactive and outreach home-based services by CIIC were beneficial to older adults and their families.

4. Discussion

In summary, this new service model suggests that CIIC bridges the gaps in existing health and social services and strengthens existing community resources such as volunteer caregiver support. To better address the experiences of service users and family care providers, services for family caregivers should include the following: (1) A wellness program for family caregivers; (2) Caregiving competence development; (3) Management competence development; (4) Ongoing support of caregiving role performance. The outcome of this model is quality of care (in terms of care for older adults and family caregiver outcomes such as family caregiver wellbeing) (Figure 1).

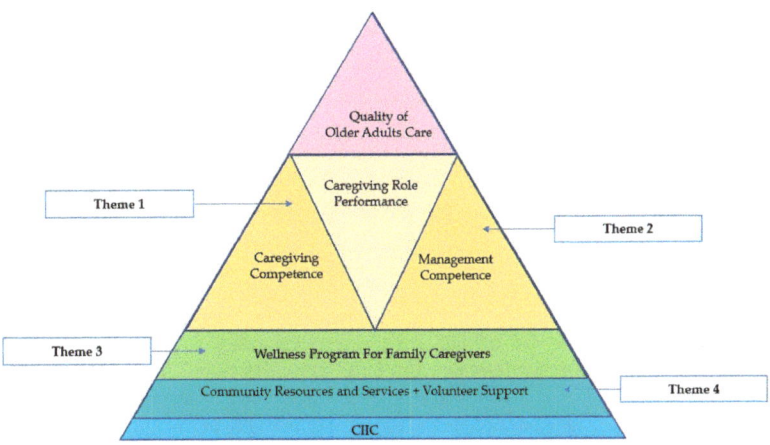

Figure 1. The Community Integrated Intermediary Care (CIIC) model, enhancing the quality of care for older adults.

Emerging themes and subthemes resulting from the qualitative analysis can be implied for CIIC as follows.

4.1. Implications of Theme 1: "Becoming a Good Caregiver" for CIIC

In consideration of the four functions of the CIIC project ((1) Screening and assessment of family burden and LTC capacity; (2) Care capacity building for family caregivers; (3) Care prevention exercise program; (4) Respite care service for families having difficulties with caregiving), we suggest that CIIC considers both principal and supplemental or other types of caregivers in capacity building. These caregivers can help share the caregiving responsibility and help offset the principal caregivers' burden and negative impacts. CIIC provides ongoing and continuous support to family caregivers and their care recipients. The support should respond to changing needs of caregiving which are developmental in nature and very dynamic across different stages of caregiving and illnesses [23,24]. Regular assessments of the needs of caregivers should also be an essential part of this ongoing support. Supports for caregivers may be guided by the developmental career of the caregiving framework.

4.2. Implications of Theme 2: "Stretching to the Limit" for CIIC

Services provided by CIIC take a family-centered approach and have dual focuses. They emphasize the needs of the care recipients and those of the caregivers. CIIC should assist health and social care providers to better understand and effectively provide family-centered services. This may be achieved through formal or informal training and workshops [24–26]. As caregiving-related stresses can be quite detrimental to the health and wellbeing of both dependent older adults and caregivers, measures to respond to their needs in a timely and adequate manner should be explored and considered by the service providers [25,27–30]. A range of innovative health and social services are suggested to be offered to caregivers. These include, and are not limited to, health promotion, illness prevention, income generation, financial assistance, counselling, social and religious activities, and respite care.

4.3. Implications of Theme 3: "Taking Care of One's Health" for CIIC

CIIC should reap the opportunity to introduce health promotion services to caregivers and families. Family caregivers are aware of staying healthy not only for themselves but also for their care recipient who is really in need of his/her help all the time. These health promotion services include the promotion of exercise activities, the introduction of a balanced diet to improve nutrition, and avoidance of substance abuse such as smoking and alcohol.

4.4. Implications of Theme 4: "Roles of CIIC in Addressing Gaps in Care and Strengthening Care Systems" for CIIC

To address the fragmentation in formal health and social services, CIIC should be involved in care management as early as possible to prevent unnecessary caregiving-related stresses and delays in accessing healthcare services. Navigation and liaison services may be considered to help bridge the gaps between different service providers [31,32]. Amidst the current lack of a designated formal care coordinator, a dedicated volunteer can be assigned and trained to serve as a care coordinator [33,34]. These volunteer coordinators work with families, social care providers, health providers, and other community organizations to ensure that older adults and families can access the needed services on a timely basis [35]. The lessons from CIIC noted that dedicated and devoted volunteers are valuable and instrumental in care management. They are advised to be equipped with the mindset, knowledge, and skills to effectively perform the assigned roles. Moreover, volunteers can be recognized as an integral part of CIIC and the wider community care systems. Their contribution to the systems should be formally and informally valued and recognized on various important community platforms. Moreover, CIIC is considered acceptable as it is a well-integrated home-based and CIIC center-based service. Alternatives to the pay-for-service approach should be explored with consideration of the abilities of the families to pay and the existing financing mechanisms of health and social services. The finding of this study to reflect the usefulness and acceptability of CIIC via qualitative evaluation may be limited by the Thai culture of consideration for others and feeling of gratitude and reciprocity. However, the strength is that our findings may form the tip of the iceberg where sustainability and maintenance of implementation are required to see the full effectiveness to provide stronger evidence for an ageing world.

5. Conclusions

Our findings supported that the experience-based design of CIIC could help family caregivers of older adults reduce caregiver burden and become good caregivers by providing ongoing and continuous support for care capacity building via a family-centered approach. In addition, CIIC also provided a respite care center to host the dependent older adults when their family caregivers are burned out or not available for caregiving temporarily. In consideration of sustainability, traditional home-based and CIIC-based services should be well integrated. A welfare-free-of-charge approach to service financing may be considered, depending on the ability of families to pay for the services. By using effective community support and local stakeholders for the provision of infrastructure for ageing care and a strong community health volunteers' network, the model of CIIC can be sustainable for healthy ageing communities in Thailand.

Author Contributions: Conceptualization, T.L. and M.N.A.; methodology, T.L., M.N.A., S.M. and T.N.N.A.; software, T.L., M.N.A., S.M. and T.N.N.A.; validation, T.L., S.M. and T.N.N.A.; formal analysis, T.L., M.N.A., S.M. and T.N.N.A.; investigation, T.N.N.A., M.N.A. and S.M.; resources, T.L., M.N.A., M.Y., Y.K. and S.S.; data curation, T.N.N.A. and S.M.; writing—original draft preparation, T.L., M.N.A., S.M. and T.N.N.A.; writing—review and editing, T.L., M.N.A., T.N.N.A., S.M., Y.K., C.A., M.Y. and S.S.; visualization, M.N.A., S.M. and T.N.N.A.; supervision, M.N.A., M.Y. and S.S.; project administration, M.N.A., S.M. and T.N.N.A.; funding acquisition, M.N.A. All authors have read and agreed to the published version of the manuscript.

Funding: This research was supported by the World Health Organization Centre for Health Development (WHO Kobe Centre—WKC: K18020). This research was partially supported by Chiang Mai University (TNNA, CA).

Institutional Review Board Statement: This study was conducted in accordance with the Declaration of Helsinki. The World Health Organization Ethical Review Committee (WHO/ERC ID; ERC.0003064, dated 7 March 2019) and Ethical Review Committee for Research in Human Subjects, Boromarajonani College of Nursing Nakhon Lampang, Praboromarajchanok under the Institute for Health Workforce Development, Ministry of Public Health, Thailand (approval number E 2562/005, dated 4 March 2019) approved the ethics of the study. It has been registered at the Thailand Clinical Trial Registry, trial registration number TCTR20190412004.

Informed Consent Statement: Written informed consent was obtained from all subjects involved in the study.

Data Availability Statement: The data presented in this study are available on request from the corresponding author.

Acknowledgments: The study participants; village health volunteers; head nurses of primary care units, Mueang Chiang Mai, Thailand; Mayor and members of Maehia municipality, Mueang Chiang Mai, Thailand; the Faculty of Science and Technology, Chiang Mai Rajabhat University, Chiang Mai, Thailand; and Japan International Cooperation Agency (JICA) are acknowledged for their contribution to and cooperation in the CIIC study.

Conflicts of Interest: The authors declare no conflict of interest. The funders had no role in the design of the study; in the collection, analyses, or interpretation of data; in the writing of the manuscript; or in the decision to publish the results.

References

1. World Health Organization. Ageing and Health. Available online: https://www.who.int/news-room/fact-sheets/detail/ageing-and-health (accessed on 2 April 2023).
2. Thailand, U. *Impact of Demographic Change in Thailand*; United Nations Population Funds; United Nations: New York, NY, USA, 2017.
3. Rudnicka, E.; Napierała, P.; Podfigurna, A.; Męczekalski, B.; Smolarczyk, R.; Grymowicz, M. The World Health Organization (WHO) approach to healthy ageing. *Maturitas* 2020, *139*, 6–11. [CrossRef] [PubMed]
4. World Health Organization. *Older Population and Health System: A Profile of Thailand*; World Health Organization: Geneva, Switzerland, 2015; Volume 10, pp. 19–36.
5. Aung, T.N.N.; Aung, M.N.; Moolphate, S.; Koyanagi, Y.; Supakankunti, S.; Yuasa, M. Caregiver Burden and Associated Factors for the Respite Care Needs among the Family Caregivers of Community Dwelling Senior Citizens in Chiang Mai, Northern Thailand. *Int. J. Environ. Res. Public Health* 2021, *18*, 5873. [CrossRef] [PubMed]
6. Aung, T.N.N.; Aung, M.N.; Moolphate, S.; Koyanagi, Y.; Ichikawa, M.; Supakankunti, S.; Yuasa, M. Estimating service demand for intermediary care at a community integrated intermediary care center among family caregivers of older adults residing in Chiang Mai, Northern Thailand. *Int. J. Environ. Res. Public Health* 2021, *18*, 6087. [CrossRef] [PubMed]
7. Knodel, J.; Teerawichitchainan, B.P.; Prachuabmoh, V.; Pothisiri, W. *The Situation of Thailand's Older Population: An Update Based on the 2014 Survey of Older Persons in Thailand*; HelpAge International: Chiang Mai, Thailand, 2015.
8. National Statistical Office. *Report on the 2017 Survey of the Older Persons in Thailand*; National Statistical Office: Bangkok, Thailand, 2018.
9. Aung, N.M.; Moolphate, S.; Yuasa, M.; Aung, N.T.N.; Koyanagi, Y.; Supakankunti, S.; Ahmad, I.; Kayano, R.; Ong, P. Community-Integrated Intermediary Care (CIIC) Service Model to Enhance Family-Based, Long-Term Care for Older People: Protocol for a Cluster Randomized Controlled Trial in Thailand. *JMIR Res. Protoc.* 2021, *10*, e20196. [CrossRef] [PubMed]
10. Aung, M.N.; Moolphate, S.; Aung, T.N.N.; Koyanagi, Y.; Kurusattra, A.; Chantaraksa, S.; Supakankunti, S.; Yuasa, M. Effectiveness of a community-integrated intermediary care (CIIC) service model to enhance family-based long-term care for Thai older adults in Chiang Mai, Thailand: A cluster-randomized controlled trial TCTR20190412004. *Health Res. Policy Syst.* 2022, *20*, 110. [CrossRef] [PubMed]
11. World Health Organization. Thailand: How a Strong Health System Fights a Pandemic. In *COVID-19: WHO's Action in Countries*; World Health Organization: Geneva, Switzerland, 2020.
12. NHS Elect. Evidence Based Design. Available online: https://www.google.com/url?sa=i&rct=j&q=&esrc=s&source=web&cd=&ved=0CAMQw7AJahcKEwjQ-f_Vqsn-AhUAAAAAHQAAAAAQAg&url=https%3A%2F%2Fnhselect.nhs.uk%2Fuploads%2Ffiles%2F1%2FEBD%2520Guide_single.pdf&psig=AOvVaw1SFybqbUZAGa5Xl3Hxrpme&ust=1682659538307495 (accessed on 27 April 2023).
13. Gustavsson, S.M.; Andersson, T. Patient involvement 2.0: Experience-based co-design supported by action research. *Action Res.* 2019, *17*, 469–491. [CrossRef]
14. Goodrich, J. Why experience-based co-design improves the patient experience. *J. Health Des.* 2018, *3*, 84–85. [CrossRef]
15. Goodyear, M.D.; Krleza-Jeric, K.; Lemmens, T. The declaration of Helsinki. *Br. Med. J. Publ. Group* 2007, *335*, 624–625. [CrossRef] [PubMed]
16. The Primary Health Care Division. *The Four-Decade Development of Primary Health Care in Thailand 1978–2014*; The War Veterans Organization of Thailand Under Royal Patronage of His Majesty The King, (Office of Printing Mill): Rajathewi Bangkok, Thailand, 2014.
17. Pitchalard, K.; Moonpanane, K.; Wimolphan, P.; Singkhorn, O.; Wongsuraprakit, S. Implementation and evaluation of the peer-training program for village health volunteers to improve chronic disease management among older adults in rural Thailand. *Int. J. Nurs. Sci.* 2022, *9*, 328–333. [CrossRef] [PubMed]
18. Doyle, L.; McCabe, C.; Keogh, B.; Brady, A.; McCann, M. An overview of the qualitative descriptive design within nursing research. *J. Res. Nurs.* 2020, *25*, 443–455. [CrossRef] [PubMed]
19. Nassaji, H. *Qualitative and Descriptive Research: Data Type Versus Data Analysis*; Sage Publications: London, UK, 2015; Volume 19, pp. 129–132.
20. Patton, M.Q. Qualitative evaluation checklist. *Eval. Checkl. Proj.* 2003, *21*, 1–13.
21. Glaser, B.G. *Doing Grounded Theory: Issues and Discussions*; Sociology Press: Mill Valley, CA, USA, 1998.
22. Lincoln, Y.S.; Guba, E.G.; Pilotta, J.J. *Naturalistic Inquiry*; Sage Publications: Beverly Hills, CA, USA, 1985; 416p.
23. Tipsuk, P. *Caring for Older Adults with Disability: Lived Experience of Family Caregivers in Rural Thailand*; Miami University: Oxford OH, USA, 2016.
24. Limpawattana, P.T.A.; Chindaprasirt, J.; Sawanyawisuth, K.; Pimporm, J. Caregivers Burden of Older Adults with Chronic Illnesses in the Community: A Cross-Sectional Study. *J. Community Health* 2013, *38*, 40–45. [CrossRef]
25. Phetsitong, R.; Vapattanawong, P.; Sunpuwan, M.; Völker, M. State of household need for caregivers and determinants of psychological burden among caregivers of older people in Thailand: An analysis from national surveys on older persons. *PLoS ONE* 2019, *14*, e0226330. [CrossRef] [PubMed]
26. Tamdee, D.; Tamdee, P.; Greiner, C.; Boonchiang, W.; Okamoto, N.; Isowa, T. Conditions of caring for the elderly and family caregiver stress in Chiang Mai, Thailand. *J. Health Res.* 2019, *33*, 138–150. [CrossRef]

27. Wongsawang, N.; Lagampan, S.; Lapvongwattana, P.; Bowers, B.J. Family caregiving for dependent older adults in Thai families. *J. Nurs. Scholarsh.* **2013**, *45*, 336–343. [CrossRef]
28. Supaporn, K.; Isaramalai, S.-A.; Khaw, T. Family Caregivers' Perceptions of Caring for Older Persons in the Palliative Care Stage at Home. *Pac. Rim Int. J. Nurs. Res.* **2022**, *26*, 161–174.
29. Gray, R.S.; Pattaravanich, U. Internal and external resources, tiredness and the subjective well-being of family caregivers of older adults: A case study from western Thailand, Southeast Asia. *Eur. J. Ageing* **2020**, *17*, 349–359. [CrossRef] [PubMed]
30. Chanprasert, P. Long-term care policy and Implementation in Thailand'. In *Coping with Rapid Population Ageing in Asia: Discussions on Long-Term Care Policy and Cross-Border Circulation of Care Workers*; Economic Research Institute for ASEAN and East Asia: Jakarta, Indonesia, 2021; pp. 36–44.
31. ADB. *Country Diagnostic Study on Long—Term Care in Thailand*; Asian Development Bank: Manila, Phillipines, 2020.
32. Vongmongkol, V.; Viriyathorn, S.; Wanwong, Y.; Wangbanjongkun, W.; Tangcharoensathien, V. Annual prevalence of unmet healthcare need in Thailand: Evidence from national household surveys between 2011 and 2019. *Int. J. Equity Health* **2021**, *20*, 1–10. [CrossRef] [PubMed]
33. Whangmahaporn, P. Characteristics of Elderly Home Care Volunteers in Western of Thailand. *Int. J. Crime Law Soc. Issues* **2018**, *5*, 382–386. [CrossRef]
34. Whangmahaporn, P. Care for the Elderly at Home Volunteers and Citizenship: Connectors to Stronger Community in Thailand. *MFU Connex. J. Humanit. Soc. Sci.* **2016**, *5*, 23–44.
35. Whangmahaporn, P. Causal factors contributing to participation in the elderly care of care-for-the-elderly-at-home volunteers in Thailand. In Proceedings of the International Conference on Ethics in Governance (ICONEG 2016), Makassar, Indonesia, 19–20 December 2016; pp. 382–386.

Disclaimer/Publisher's Note: The statements, opinions and data contained in all publications are solely those of the individual author(s) and contributor(s) and not of MDPI and/or the editor(s). MDPI and/or the editor(s) disclaim responsibility for any injury to people or property resulting from any ideas, methods, instructions or products referred to in the content.

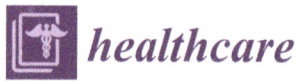

Article

Outcomes of a Self-Management Program for People with Non-Communicable Diseases in the Context of COVID-19

Rodrigo Cesar León Hernández [1,*], Jorge Luis Arriaga Martínez [2], Martha Arely Hernández Del Angel [2], Isabel Peñarrieta de Córdova [2], Virginia Solís Solís [3] and María Elena Velásquez Salinas [4]

1. Consejo Nacional de Humanidades Ciencias y Tecnologías CONAHCYT, Mexico City 03940, Mexico
2. Facultad de Enfermería Tampico, Universidad Autónoma de Tamaulipas, Centro Universitario Tampico-Madero, Tampico 89339, Mexico; jorge.arriaga@uat.edu.mx (J.L.A.M.); marthahdz@docentes.uat.edu.mx (M.A.H.D.A.); pcordoba@docentes.uat.edu.mx (I.P.d.C.)
3. Ministerio de Salud de Perú, Lima 15046, Peru; vsoliss@minsa.gob.pe
4. Dirección de Redes Integradas de Salud Lima Centro, Ministerio de Salud de Perú, Lima 15001, Peru; discapacidad@dirislimacentro.gob.pe
* Correspondence: rcleonhe@conahcyt.mx; Tel.: +52-833-106-9209

Abstract: Objective: To evaluate the effectiveness of the online version of the Chronic Disease Self-Management Program (CDSMP) on physical activity and depressive symptoms in individuals with non-communicable diseases (NCDs) in Mexico and Peru during the COVID-19 pandemic. Materials and Methods: Quasi-experimental study with a non-probability sample of 114 people with NCDs, recruited by invitation in Mexico and by convenience in Peru. The participants were assigned to intervention (n = 85) and control (n = 29) groups. The Personal Health Questionnaire (PHQ-8) and the Physical Activity Scale were used to assess the outcomes. Measurements were taken before and after the intervention. The CDSMP comprises six sessions that take place once per week and last 2.5 h each. Results: The intervention group showed a significant reduction in depressive symptoms and an increase in physical activity (PA) at the end of the program. In contrast, the control group showed no significant improvement in depression and presented a significant decrease in PA.

Keywords: depression; physical activity; self-management; non-communicable diseases

Citation: Hernández, R.C.L.; Martínez, J.L.A.; Del Angel, M.A.H.; de Córdova, I.P.; Solís, V.S.; Salinas, M.E.V. Outcomes of a Self-Management Program for People with Non-Communicable Diseases in the Context of COVID-19. Healthcare 2024, 12, 1668. https://doi.org/10.3390/healthcare12161668

Academic Editor: Hidetaka Hamasaki

Received: 12 July 2024
Revised: 8 August 2024
Accepted: 17 August 2024
Published: 21 August 2024

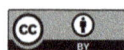

Copyright: © 2024 by the authors. Licensee MDPI, Basel, Switzerland. This article is an open access article distributed under the terms and conditions of the Creative Commons Attribution (CC BY) license (https://creativecommons.org/licenses/by/4.0/).

1. Introduction

In the changing global health landscape, chronic or non-communicable diseases (NCDs) represent one of the greatest challenges of the 21st century. According to data from the World Health Organization (WHO), approximately 74% of global deaths are attributable to these diseases, which are primarily cardiovascular diseases, cancer, chronic respiratory diseases, and diabetes [1]. In addition to representing a direct threat to life, these diseases can also give rise to a range of psychological complications, with depression being a particularly prevalent consequence [2]. The epidemiological landscape in low- and middle-income countries is comparable. In Mexico, NCDs account for approximately 75% of deaths, with depression specifically affecting around 9% of the adult population. An increase in major depression cases has been observed among adolescents and young adults [3]. Similarly, these diseases pose a significant burden on public health in Peru, contributing to 73% of total deaths. Recent studies indicate that approximately 7% of adult Peruvians suffer from depression, with a notable rise in cases during and after the COVID-19 pandemic [4].

The interaction between NCDs and depression is "a two-way street" [5], i.e., while living with a chronic disease may increase the risk of developing depression, the incidence of depression also increases as these diseases accumulate [6]. The evidence suggests that 30% of people with an NCD suffer from depression, and this figure rises to 41% in the presence of multimorbidity, the presence of three or more diseases [7]. Likewise, depression can aggravate the symptoms of an NCD, hinder self-care, and worsen clinical outcomes [3,8,9]. It can also impede treatment follow-up and proper care of NCDs, increasing the risk of multiple complications [9] and their duration [5]. Furthermore, depression can ultimately impair an individual's capacity to engage in daily activities and negatively impact their quality of life [9,10].

The management of NCDs encompasses three primary strategies: physiological support, risk-factor education, and regular physical activity [11]. In this sense, the scientific literature supports that regular physical activity (PA) is an effective treatment for these diseases [6,12–14]. However, a lack of PA also has detrimental effects on health; people who are physically inactive have an increased risk of mortality [13,15]. They are also twice as likely to experience depressive symptoms [16].

On the one hand, some studies have investigated the relationship between depression and PA, documenting that regular exercise not only benefits physical fitness but also plays a crucial role in improving the mental and emotional state of people living with NCDs [12,16]; one of the most notable findings is that adults who comply with regular PA guidelines have lower levels of depression [14,16–18]. The implementation of PA has been demonstrated to enhance a number of domains that are adversely affected by NCDs. These include body weight, fatigue, mental well-being, muscle and bone strength, physical capacity, and quality of life [11]. On the other hand, physical inactivity has been found to be associated with an increased risk of depression [16,19], particularly in women. [20].

Against this backdrop, there is a need for multimodal therapeutic approaches to address the problem of NCDs. Self-management programs, which aim to equip patients with skills and tools to manage their health, are a promising strategy. There is a large body of empirical evidence supporting the effectiveness of chronic disease self-management programs (CDSMPs or Tomando Control de su Salud (Spanish version)) across diverse formats, settings, and populations [21,22]. This research has evaluated outcomes that include improvements in quality of life [23–25], adherence [23,26,27], and reductions in hospitalizations and physician visits [24,28–30], which are promising for the improvement of depression and anxiety [21].

In Mexico, the CDSMP program has shown similar results in reducing depression and stress, improving social activity limitation, perception of quality of life, and communication with physicians. Concurrently, an augmentation in the level of physical activity, adherence to medical appointments, and self-management practice have been documented [31]. Finally, the CDSM program has demonstrated its effectiveness when implemented virtually. Participants in the program experienced significant improvements in self-efficacy, reduced pain and fatigue, and better chronic symptom management [32]. Additionally, there was a decrease in emergency room visits and hospitalizations [33]. During the COVID-19 pandemic, studies conducted in New York [34] and Washington [35] reported similar results with the virtual modality, including significant improvements in self-efficacy, a notable reduction in HbA1c levels and depression, and an increase in physical activity and healthy eating habits. In Mexico and Peru, enhancements in self-efficacy, disease knowledge, treatment adherence, and symptom management were also observed [36].

The literature presented above confirms the health problem represented by NCDs. It also provides evidence of the effectiveness of the CDSMP, particularly on the variables of PA and depression. However, there is a lack of studies on the impact of the program in the Latin American region, especially during the COVID-19 pandemic, which was a complicated historical moment for people living with such diseases.

In the context of the pandemic, people with NCDs were considered a vulnerable group, as they were more susceptible to infection or death due to the virus [37] and to developing severe complications from COVID-19 [38–40]. Furthermore, indirect effects of COVID-19 on the treatment and self-management of people with NCDs were found. For example, social distancing measures affected the attendance of visits to specialists and the lack of production of NCD drugs [41], as well as the effects of unemployment and lack of access to social security [42].

It is also known that the COVID-19 pandemic caused drastic changes in daily life, with confinement and social distancing limiting the usual physical activities [40]. These limitations created an environment in which maintaining adequate levels of PA could be challenging and highlighted the need to deliver programs remotely, safely, and efficiently [37,43]. Given this situation, it became imperative to adapt and implement virtual programs [44] that promote PA and a healthy mental state.

In view of the serious problem of NCDs and their impact on PA and mental health, which were exacerbated during the pandemic, as well as evidence of the positive results of the aforementioned program, the aim of the present study was to evaluate the effectiveness of the online version of the CDSMP program on physical activity and depressive symptoms in people with NCDs in Mexico and Peru during the COVID-19 pandemic.

2. Materials and Methods

2.1. Participants

The non-probabilistic initial sample consisted of 132 people with non-communicable diseases. The sampling was mixed: by invitation in Mexico and by convenience in Peru. Those with a diagnosis of NCD of more than 3 months at the time of the study were included. Those under 18 years of age and those who did not respond to all the instruments were excluded. The participants were consecutively assigned to intervention and control groups; the final sample consisted of 114 participants: intervention group (n = 85) and control group (n = 29). The process for forming the study sample is shown in Figure 1. The design of this study was quasi-experimental with independent (intervention and control) and repeated (pretest–posttest) measurements.

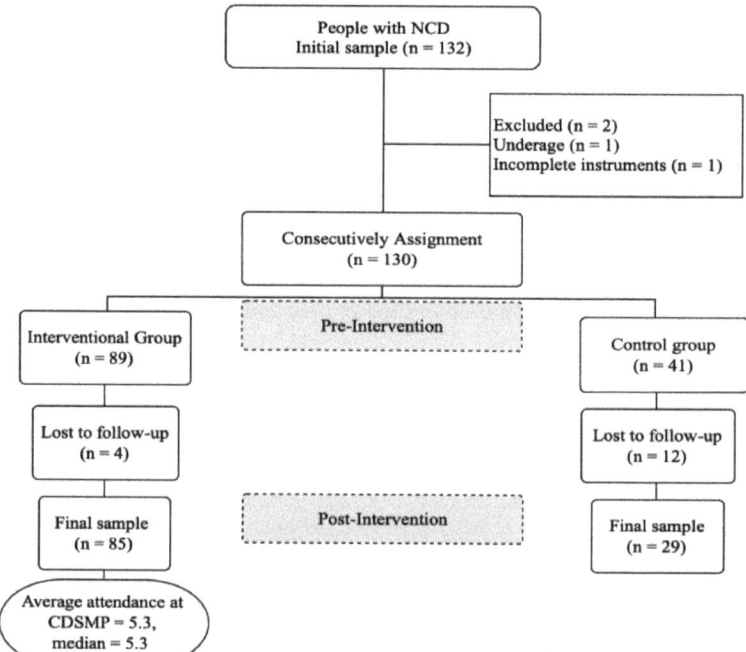

Figure 1. Study sample.

2.2. Measuring Instruments

The Personal Health Questionnaire (PHQ) was used to measure depression. The version validated in Mexico consists of 8 items and a Likert-type scale with 4 options (from 0 points = no day to 3 = almost every day). An overall score is obtained by summing the responses and is categorized into no depressive symptoms, 0–4 points; mild symptoms, 5–9; moderate symptoms, 10–14; severe symptoms, 15–19; and very severe symptoms, 20–24 points. The internal consistency was $\alpha = 0.78$ [45]. Physical activity was measured using the Lorig et al. scale [46], which consists of 6 items assessing the frequency of exercise in minutes per week, with 5 response options ranging from 0 = none to 4 = more than 3 h. It is interpreted using the average score when the items are added together. Its validation in Mexico showed an internal consistency of $\alpha = 0.62$ and a test–retest reliability = 0.72 [45].

2.3. Procedures

Initially, approval for the use of the CDSMP program was obtained from authorities at the Faculty of Nursing, Tampico-Universidad Autónoma de Tamaulipas, Mexico, and the National Institute of Neoplastic Diseases (INEN), Peru. Trained facilitators or leaders then recruited people with NCDs. In Mexico, a call for applications was disseminated through social networks during the second half of 2021. In Peru, the INEN worker leaders invited the users of the institute to participate in the study during the first semester of 2022. Assignment to the intervention and control groups was non-randomized. Before and after taking part in the program, the instruments were applied (pretest and posttest measurements), which were automated using the Google Forms platform (https://workspace.google.com/products/forms/). The posttest was applied at the end of the sixth session in the intervention groups and the same day in the controls.

The CDSMP program, an online format, consists of six sessions of 2.5 h each, meeting once a week, and is facilitated by two people who have been previously trained and certified by Stanford University. Its content addresses topics related to healthy eating, exercise, decision-making, symptoms such as sleep, pain, and fatigue, managing difficult emotions, problem-solving, communication skills, and goal setting [47].

2.4. Ethical Considerations

This study is part of a project funded by the Consejo Nacional de Humanidades Ciencias y Tecnologías, CF-2023-G-1394, entitled "Self-Management Strategies to Improve the Health of Persons with Chronic Illness and Family Caregivers. A Networked Work". It was approved by the Research Ethics Committee of the Tampico Nursing School, Universidad Autónoma de Tamaulipas, registration number FET/CI/2023/002, and by the Institutional Research Ethics Committee of INEN, letter No. 149-2020-CIEI/INEN. The study adhered to the guidelines established in the Regulations of the General Health Law on Health Research in Mexico [48] and the Helsinki Declaration [49].

2.5. Statistical Analysis

Frequencies, percentages, and means and standard deviations were used to describe the characteristics of the study sample. The Kolmogorov–Smirnov test was used to determine the normality criteria of the variables, which showed significant results ($p < 0.05$): Nonparametric inferential tests were used for the above: the Mann–Whitney U and Wilcoxon tests. The analyses were performed using the Statistical Package for the Social Sciences (SPSS-25).

3. Results

The sociodemographic characteristics show that 83.3% of the participants were female. The mean age was 58.8, with a standard deviation of 11.5. The predominant nationality was Peruvian (81.6%), marital status was married (53.4%), and the most frequent NCD reported by participants was cancer (28%) (see Table 1).

Table 1. Sociodemographic characteristics.

n = 114	f	%
Gender		
Female	95	83.3
Male	19	16.7
Nationality		
Perú	93	81.6
México	21	18.4
Marital status		
Married	61	53.4
Divorced	7	6.1
Single	27	23.6
Widower	19	16.9
First NCD reported		
Cancer	28	36.8
Diabetes	18	23.7
Hypertension	11	14.5
Other NCDs reported	19	25.0
Total =	114	100%

Note: f = frequencies, % = percentages.

The results of the comparison test between the intervention and control groups (Mann–Whitney U) show that there were no significant differences ($p > 0.05$) in the depression and PA variables in the pretest measure, therefore, the groups were equal before starting the intervention. However, in the posttest measure, significant differences were detected in both variables ($p < 0.001$) (see Table 2).

Table 2. Comparison between groups (intervention and control) in pretest–posttest measures.

Inter-Subjects	Intervention Groups (n = 85)			Control Groups (n = 29)			Sig.
	Mean Rank	Mean (SD)	Median	Mean Rank	Mean (SD)	Median	
Depression pretest	54.95	6.01 (5.0)	3	63.23	6.04 (4.9)	4.5	0.243
Physical activity pretest	57.50	120.4 (126.1)	75	57.52	133.4 (158.1)	60	0.973
Depression posttest	51.51	3.26 (4.1)	1	75.07	5.86 (4.3)	6	<0.001
Physical activity posttest	66.68	160.4 (124.2)	135	30.60	53.8 (62.9)	30	<0.001

Note: n = sample, Sig. = significance, SD = standard deviation.

To achieve the research objective, the Wilcoxon signed-rank test was applied. As can be seen in Table 2, significant results ($p < 0.05$) were seen in the intervention group for the two research variables (see Table 3).

Table 3. Pretest–posttest depression and physical activity, intervention groups.

Intra-Subjects n = 85	Mean Rank		Mean (SD)		Median		Sig.
	Positive	Negative	Pretest	Posttest	Pretest	Posttest	
Depression (R 0–24)	25.44	34.23	6.01 (5.0)	3.26 (4.1)	3	1	<0.001
Physical activity (R 0–1080)	39.21	43.50	120.4 (126.1)	160.4 (124.2)	75	135	0.006

Note: n = sample, Sig. = significance, SD = standard deviation, R = range.

With respect to the control group, the results of the analysis show statistically significant differences in PA ($p = 0.003$) but not in depression (see Table 4).

Table 4. Pretest-posttest depression and physical activity, control groups.

Pretest–Posttest n = 29	Mean Rank		Mean (SD)		Median		Sig.
	Positive	Negative	Pretest	Posttest	Pretest	Posttest	
Depression (R 0–24)	13.55	11.62	6.04 (4.9)	5.86 (4.3)	4.5	6	0.977
Physical activity (R 0–1080)	6.08	13.53	133.4 (158.1)	53.8 (62.9)	60	30	0.003

Note: n = sample, Sig. = significance, SD = standard deviation, R = range.

In order to clarify the direction of the changes of interest in the intervention group and the control group, graphs were plotted using the value of the median, before (pretest) and after (posttest) the intervention. In Figure 2, it can be seen that the intervention group showed a significant improvement in reducing depression, while the control group worsened during the same period.

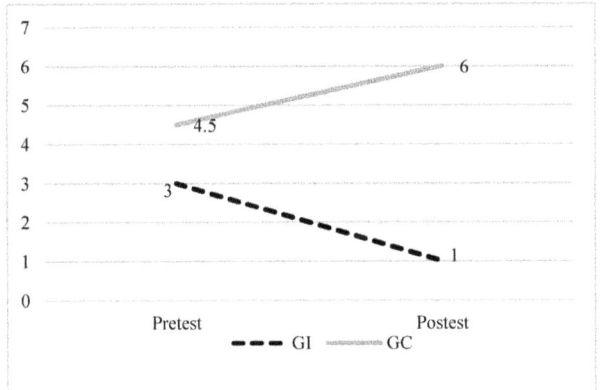

Figure 2. Results of the CDSMP program for the depression variable. Note: pretest and posttest medians for depression in the intervention (dashed line) and control groups (solid line).

Figure 3 shows a marked improvement in the PA level of the intervention group after the program, increasing from 75 to 135 min of exercise, in contrast to the control group, which experienced a reduction in activity level in the same time frame.

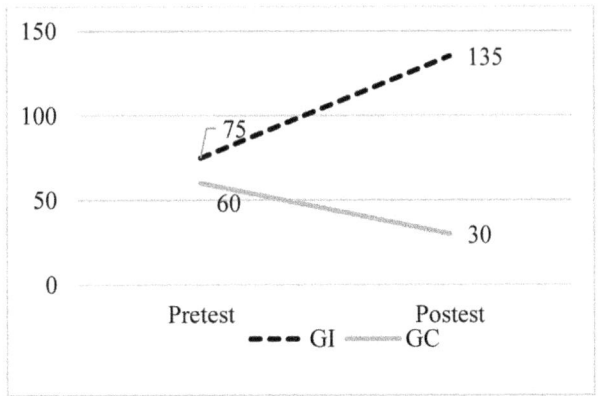

Figure 3. CDSMP program results for the physical activity variable. Note: pretest and posttest medians in the physical activity variable of the intervention (dashed line) and control groups (solid line).

4. Discussion

The objective of this study was to evaluate the efficacy of the online version of the CDSMP program on physical activity and depressive symptoms in people with NCDs in Mexico and Peru during the COVID-19 pandemic. In response to the above, the results indicate significant improvements in PA and a reduction in depressive symptoms in the intervention group at the end of the CDSMP program. In contrast, the control group showed negative results in both variables, which were significant in the case of PA. In other words, users with NCDs who did not participate in the program during the pandemic period significantly decreased their PA practice. These findings demonstrate the efficacy of the online CDSMP to improve these two key aspects of health in individuals with NCDs, which, on the one hand, are considered an effective treatment for these diseases [6,12–14,20], and on the other hand, interact in a reciprocal manner leading to a deterioration in health [5,6,8–10].

The improvement in PA and the decrease in depression reflect results similar to previous studies [23–25,34], which also documented benefits in quality of life and adherence to post-intervention treatment. However, these findings provide new evidence of the effects of the CDSMP program in Latin American contexts, where there is a paucity of studies documenting these effects. In this regard, only the study by Peñarrieta et al. [31], in which they applied the same program in a face-to-face format, with a sample of people with NCD in Mexico, reported similar results with benefits in PA and depression at 3 and 6 months, compared with the control group. It should be noted that no empirical evidence was detected that reports any negative effects of the CDSMP program on PA and depression, therefore, the results of this study are similar to the international literature.

In regard to the control group, a negative and significant effect on PA was discerned. This confirms the findings of some authors who found that during the social distancing and health restrictions adopted during the pandemic, PA could be affected or limited, underscoring the importance of implementing distance programs [37,43,50]. These contributed to reducing the complications to which people with NCD were exposed [37–40], such as the increased risk of mortality and depressive symptoms [13,15,16].

With regard to the depression variable, the contrast between the results observed in the intervention and control groups (see Figure 2) allows us to affirm that the CDSMP program can be an extremely important tool, since it has been documented that depression interferes with self-care and treatment follow-up, in addition to worsening clinical outcomes, quality of life, and affecting daily activities [5,8–10].

In addition, the favorable results of the CDSMP online format could have a positive impact on some of the problems that were accentuated during the pandemic, such as non-attendance at specialist consultations or lack of access to social security [41,42]. Therefore, it is suggested to continue disseminating the program and provide evidence to support its efficacy in different Latin American countries, as well as its benefits in face-to-face and virtual formats. It is also suggested that the CDSMP be proposed among the health-related public policies of Mexico and Peru since there is evidence supporting the program's contribution to reducing or postponing negative consequences on the health of people with NCDs.

With reference to the limitations of this study, the drawbacks derived from the social distancing that occurred during the COVID-19 pandemic are highlighted, which made it difficult to form the study sample. Thus, the non-randomization in the assignment to the intervention and control groups was also a limitation; however, the equality test between groups in the pretest measure ensured its initial equivalence. Finally, the absence of follow up measures is also an important limitation, so it is suggested to perform measurements at 6 and 12 months in subsequent studies.

5. Conclusions

The TCS program in an online format proved to be an effective tool for improving physical activity and reducing depression in people with NCDs in Mexico and Peru particularly in the context of the pandemic, when access to face-to-face health facilities was limited. Therefore, for future research, it is suggested to replicate self-management programs in virtual formats, as well as to carry out medium- and long-term evaluations, to address public health challenges in developing countries.

In conclusion, the results of this work contribute to the body of evidence supporting the CDSPM program worldwide. The practical implications are that the online CDSPM represents a valuable tool to combat NCDs in Latin American countries such as Peru and Mexico, where epidemiological indicators position them as serious health problems and health systems lack the capacity to provide adequate face-to-face services.

Author Contributions: Conceptualization, J.L.A.M. and M.A.H.D.A.; methodology, R.C.L.H. and V.S.S.; formal analysis, R.C.L.H. and I.P.d.C.; investigation, M.E.V.S. and I.P.d.C.; data curation, R.C.L.H. and I.P.d.C.; writing—original draft preparation, J.L.A.M. and M.A.H.D.A.; writing—review and editing, V.S.S. and M.E.V.S.; supervision, R.C.L.H. and I.P.d.C.; funding acquisition, R.C.L.H. All authors have read and agreed to the published version of the manuscript.

Funding: This work is the result of the federal research project (CF-2023-G-1394) entitled: "Estrategias de automanejo para mejorar la salud de personas con enfermedades crónicas y cuidadores familiares. Un trabajo en Red". Consejo Nacional de Humanidades, Ciencias y Tecnologías (CONAHCYT). The source of federal funds did not impact the study design, data collection, analysis, interpretation, or manuscript writing.

Institutional Review Board Statement: The study was conducted according to the guidelines of the Declaration of Helsinki and approved by the Research Ethics Committee of the Tampico Nursing School, Universidad Autónoma de Tamaulipas, registration number FET/CI/2023/002 (approved on 5 July 2023) and by the Institutional Research Ethics Committee of INEN, letter No. 149-2020-CIEI/INEN (approved on 18 October 2021).

Informed Consent Statement: Informed consent was obtained from all the subjects involved in the study.

Data Availability Statement: The datasets used during the current study are available from the corresponding author upon reasonable request.

Acknowledgments: The authors thank Red Temática de Automanejo en Enfermedades Crónicas. (Chronic Diseases Self-Management Thematic Network).

Conflicts of Interest: The authors declare no conflicts of interest.

References

1. Organización Mundial de la Salud Enfermedades no Transmisibles. Fact-Sheets. Available online: https://www.who.int/es/news-room/fact-sheets/detail/noncommunicable-diseases (accessed on 14 April 2024).
2. Ma, Y.; Xiang, Q.; Yan, C.; Liao, H.; Wang, J. Relationship between chronic diseases and depression: The mediating effect of pain. *BMC Psychiatry* **2021**, *21*, 436. [CrossRef] [PubMed]
3. de Salud, S. Panorama Epidemiológico de las Enfermedades No Transmisibles en México [Internet]. gob.mx. Available online: https://www.gob.mx/salud/documentos/panorama-epidemiologico-de-las-enfermedades-no-transmisibles-en-mexico-269304 (accessed on 1 August 2024).
4. CEPLAN. Observatorio Nacional de Prospectiva. Gob.pe. Available online: https://observatorio.ceplan.gob.pe/ficha/t17 (accessed on 1 August 2024).
5. Zavala, G.A.; Jennings, H.M.; Afaq, S.; Alam, A.; Ahmed, N.; Aslam, F.; Arsh, A.; Coales, K.; Ekers, D.; Nabi, M.; et al. Effectiveness and implementation of psychological interventions for depression in people with non-communicable diseases in South Asia: Systematic review and meta-analysis. *Int. J. Ment. Health* **2023**, *52*, 260–284. [CrossRef]
6. Andrade-Lima, A.; Werneck, A.O.; Szwarcwald, C.L.; Schuch, F.B.; Stubbs, B.; Bastos, A.A.; Silva, D.R. The role of physical activity in the association between multimorbidity and depressive symptoms: Data from 60,202 adults from the Brazilian National Health Survey. *J. Psychosom. Res.* **2020**, *134*, 110122. [CrossRef] [PubMed]
7. Zhou, P.; Wang, S.; Yan, Y.; Lu, Q.; Pei, J.; Guo, W.; Yang, X.; Li, Y. Association between chronic diseases and depression in the middle-aged and older adult Chinese population—A seven-year follow-up study based on CHARLS. *Front. Public Health* **2023**, *11*, 1176669. [CrossRef]
8. Bobo, W.V.; Grossardt, B.R.; Virani, S.; Sauver, J.L.S.; Boyd, C.M.; Rocca, W.A. Association of Depression and Anxiety With the Accumulation of Chronic Conditions. *JAMA Netw. Open* **2022**, *5*, E229817. [CrossRef] [PubMed]

9. Herrera, P.A.; Campos-Romero, S.; Szabo, W.; Martínez, P.; Guajardo, V.; Rojas, G. Understanding the Relationship between Depression and Chronic Diseases Such as Diabetes and Hypertension: A Grounded Theory Study. *Int. J. Environ. Res. Public Health* **2021**, *18*, 12130. [CrossRef] [PubMed]
10. National Institute of Mental Health Understanding the Link Between Chronic Disease and Depression. NIH Publication No. 24-MH-8015. Available online: https://www.nimh.nih.gov/health/publications/chronic-illness-mental-health (accessed on 6 June 2024).
11. Pérez-Gisbert, L.; Torres-Sánchez, I.; Ortiz-Rubio, A.; Calvache-Mateo, A.; López-López, L.; Cabrera-Martos, I.; Valenza, M.C. Effects of the COVID-19 pandemic on physical activity in chronic diseases: A systematic review and meta-analysis. *Int. J. Environ. Res. Public Health* **2021**, *18*, 12278. [CrossRef]
12. Mahindru, A.; Patil, P.; Agrawal, V. Role of Physical Activity on Mental Health and Well-Being: A Review. *Cureus* **2023**, *15*, e33475. [CrossRef]
13. Posadzki, P.; Pieper, D.; Bajpai, R.; Makaruk, H.; Könsgen, N.; Neuhaus, A.L.; Semwal, M. Exercise/physical activity and health outcomes: An overview of Cochrane systematic reviews. *BMC Public Health* **2020**, *20*, 1724. [CrossRef]
14. Adamson, B.C.; Yang, Y.; Motl, R.W. Association between compliance with physical activity guidelines, sedentary behavior and depressive symptoms. *Prev. Med.* **2016**, *91*, 152–157. [CrossRef]
15. Organización Mundial de la Salud Estadísticas Sanitarias Mundiales 2020: Monitoreando la salud para los ODS, Objetivo de Desarrollo Sostenible. 9789240011953. Available online: https://www.who.int/es/publications/i/item/9789240005105 (accessed on 6 June 2024).
16. Gao, Z.; Lee, J.E. Promoting Physical Activity and Reducing Sedentary Behavior to Prevent Chronic Diseases during the COVID Pandemic and Beyond. *J. Clin. Med.* **2022**, *11*, 4666. [CrossRef]
17. Pearce, M.; Garcia, L.; Abbas, A.; Strain, T.; Schuch, F.B.; Golubic, R.; Kelly, P.; Khan, S.; Utukuri, M.; Laird, Y.; et al. Association Between Physical Activity and Risk of Depression A Systematic Review and Meta-analysis Supplemental content. *JAMA Psychiatry* **2022**, *79*, 550–559. [CrossRef]
18. Rietz, M.; Lehr, A.; Mino, E.; Lang, A.; Szczerba, E.; Schiemann, T.; Herder, C.; Saatmann, N.; Geidl, W.; Barbaresko, J.; et al. Physical Activity and Risk of Major Diabetes-Related Complications in Individuals with Diabetes: A Systematic Review and Meta-Analysis of Observational Studies. *Diabetes Care* **2022**, *45*, 3101–3111. [CrossRef]
19. Casanova, F.; O'Loughlin, J.; Karageorgiou, V.; Beaumont, R.N.; Bowden, J.; Wood, A.R.; Tyrrell, J. Effects of physical activity and sedentary time on depression, anxiety and well-being: A bidirectional Mendelian randomisation study. *BMC Med.* **2023**, *21*, 501. [CrossRef] [PubMed]
20. Gomes, R.d.S.; Barbosa, A.R.; Meneghini, V.; Confortin, S.C.; D'orsi, E.; Rech, C.R. Association between chronic diseases, multimorbidity and insufficient physical activity among older adults in southern Brazil: A cross-sectional study. *Sao Paulo Med. J.* **2020**, *138*, 545–553. [CrossRef]
21. Brahim, L.O.; Lambert, S.D.; Feeley, N.; Coumoundouros, C.; Schaffler, J.; McCusker, J.; Moodie, E.E.M.; Kayser, J.; Kolne, K.; Belzile, E.; et al. The effects of self-management interventions on depressive symptoms in adults with chronic physical disease(s) experiencing depressive symptomatology: A systematic review and meta-analysis. *BMC Psychiatry* **2021**, *21*, 584. [CrossRef]
22. Mansoor, K.; Khuwaja, H.M.A. The effectiveness of a chronic Disease Self-Management Program for elderly people: A systematic review. *Elder. Health J.* **2020**, *6*, 51–63. [CrossRef]
23. Salvatore, A.L.; Ahn, S.; Jiang, L.; Lorig, K.; Ory, M.G. National study of chronic disease self-management: 6-month and 12-month findings among cancer survivors and non-cancer survivors. *Psychooncology* **2015**, *24*, 1714–1722. [CrossRef] [PubMed]
24. Hevey, D.; O'Raghallaigh, J.W.; O'Doherty, V.; Lonergan, K.; Heffernan, M.; Lunt, V.; Mulhern, S.; Lowry, D.; Larkin, N.; McSharry, K.; et al. Pre-post effectiveness evaluation of Chronic Disease Self-Management Program (CDSMP) participation on health, well-being and health service utilization. *Chronic Illn.* **2020**, *16*, 146–158. [CrossRef]
25. Campbell, D.; O'raghallaigh, J.W.; O'doherty, V.; Lunt, V.; Lowry, D.; Mulhern, S.; Lonergan, K.; McSharry, K.; Lynnott, J.; Forry, M.; et al. Investigating the impact of a chronic disease self-management programme on depression and quality of life scores in an Irish sample. *Psychol. Health Med.* **2022**, *27*, 1609–1617. [CrossRef]
26. Lee, S.; Jiang, L.; Dowdy, D.; Hong, Y.A.; Ory, M.G. Effects of the Chronic Disease Self-Management Program on medication adherence among older adults. *Transl. Behav. Med.* **2019**, *9*, 380–388. [CrossRef]
27. Hoong, J.M.; Koh, H.A.; Wong, K.; Lee, H.H. Effects of a community-based chronic disease self-management programme on chronic disease patients in Singapore. *Chronic Illn.* **2022**, *19*, 434–443. [CrossRef] [PubMed]
28. Tan, S.S.; Pisano, M.M.; Boone, A.L.; Baker, G.; Pers, Y.-M.; Pilotto, A.; Valsecchi, V.; Zora, S.; Zhang, X.; Fierloos, I.; et al. Evaluation Design of EFFICHRONIC: The Chronic Disease Self-Management Programme (CDSMP) Intervention for Citizens with a Low Socioeconomic Position. *Int. J. Environ. Res. Public Health* **2019**, *16*, 1883. [CrossRef] [PubMed]
29. Ferretti, L.A.; McCallion, P. Translating the Chronic Disease Self-Management Program for Community-Dwelling Adults With Developmental Disabilities. *J. Aging Health* **2019**, *31*, 22S–38S. [CrossRef]
30. Muscat, D.M.; Song, W.; Cvejic, E.; Ting, J.H.C.; Medlin, J.; Nutbeam, D. The Impact of the Chronic Disease Self-Management Program on Health Literacy: A Pre-Post Study Using a Multi-Dimensional Health Literacy Instrument. *Int. J. Environ. Res. Public Health* **2019**, *17*, 58. [CrossRef] [PubMed]
31. de Córdova, M.I.P.; Leon, R.; Gutierrez, T.; Mier, N.; Banda, O.; Delabra, M. Effectiveness of a chronic disease self-management program in Mexico: A randomized controlled study. *J. Nurs. Educ. Pr.* **2017**, *7*, 87–94. [CrossRef]

32. Lorig, K.R.; Ritter, P.L.; Laurent, D.D.; Plant, K. Internet-based chronic disease self-management: A randomized trial. *Med. Care* **2006**, *44*, 964–971. [CrossRef]
33. Lorig, K.; Ritter, P.L.; Plant, K.; Laurent, D.D.; Kelly, P.; Rowe, S. The South Australia health chronic disease self-management internet trial. *Health Educ. Behav.* **2013**, *40*, 67–77. [CrossRef]
34. Brunner, W.M.; Pullyblank, K.; Scribani, M.B.; Krupa, N.; Wyckoff, L. Remote delivery of self-management education workshops for adults with chronic pain, 2020–2021. *Chronic Illn.* **2024**, *20*, 360–368. [CrossRef]
35. Burciaga, J.J.R. Lessons learned from online chronic disease self-management program during COVID-19 pandemic [Internet]. *Res. Sq.* **2023**. Version 1. [CrossRef]
36. Hernández, R.C.L.; Martínez, J.L.A.; Pérez, A.C.R.; de Córdova, M.I.P.; Mendoza, M.F.C.; Campos, G.V. Resultados de 'Tomando Control de su Salud' online, en personas con enfermedades no transmisibles de México y Perú durante COVID-19. *Horiz. Enferm.* **2023**, 60–67. [CrossRef]
37. Wang, H.; Yuan, X.; Wang, J.; Sun, C.; Wang, G. Telemedicine maybe an effective solution for management of chronic disease during the COVID-19 epidemic. *Prim. Health Care Res. Dev.* **2021**, *22*, e48. [CrossRef]
38. Muhamad, S.-A.; Ugusman, A.; Kumar, J.; Skiba, D.; Hamid, A.A.; Aminuddin, A. COVID-19 and Hypertension: The What, the Why, and the How. *Front. Physiol.* **2021**, *12*, 665064. [CrossRef] [PubMed]
39. Azarpazhooh, M.R.; Morovatdar, N.; Avan, A.; Phan, T.G.; Divani, A.A.; Yassi, N.; Stranges, S.; Silver, B.; Biller, J.; Belasi, M.T.; et al. COVID-19 pandemic and burden of non-communicable diseases: An ecological study on data of 185 countries. *J. Stroke Cerebrovasc. Dis.* **2020**, *29*, 105089. [CrossRef] [PubMed]
40. Ushigome, E.; Hamaguchi, M.; Sudo, K.; Kitagawa, N.; Kondo, Y.; Imai, D.; Hattori, T.; Matsui, T.; Yamazaki, M.; Sawa, T.; et al. Impact of untreated diabetes and COVID-19-related diabetes on severe COVID-19. *Heliyon* **2022**, *8*, e08801. [CrossRef] [PubMed]
41. Ghotbi, T.; Salami, J.; Kalteh, E.A.; Ghelichi-Ghojogh, M. Self-management of patients with chronic diseases during COVID19: A narrative review. *J. Prev. Med. Hyg.* **2021**, *62*, E814–E821. [CrossRef] [PubMed]
42. Hartmann-Boyce, J.; Morris, E.; Goyder, C.; Kinton, J.; Perring, J.; Nunan, D.; Mahtani, K.; Buse, J.B.; Del Prato, S.; Ji, L.; et al. Diabetes and COVID-19: Risks, Management, and Learnings From Other National Disasters. *Diabetes Care* **2020**, *43*, 1695–1703. [CrossRef]
43. Sanchez-Ramirez, D.C.; Pol, M.; Loewen, H.; Choukou, M.-A. Effect of telemonitoring and telerehabilitation on physical activity, exercise capacity, health-related quality of life and healthcare use in patients with chronic lung diseases or COVID-19: A scoping review. *J. Telemed. Telecare* **2022**, 1357633X221122124. [CrossRef] [PubMed]
44. Gray, S.M.; Franke, T.; Sims-Gould, J.; McKay, H.A. Rapidly adapting an effective health promoting intervention for older adults—Choose to move—For virtual delivery during the COVID-19 pandemic. *BMC Public Health* **2022**, *22*, 1172. [CrossRef]
45. Hernández, R.C.L.; de Córdova, M.I.P.; Gómez, T.G. Validación de instrumentos de indicadores de salud y psicosociales. Red de automanejo de enfermedades crónicas. In *Estrategias de Aprendizaje en Cronicidad*, 1st ed.; Consejo de Publicaciones UAT, Ed.; Colofón: Ciudad de México, Mexico, 2019; pp. 65–84. Available online: https://www.researchgate.net/publication/358906879_Validacion_de_instrumentos_de_indicadores_de_salud_y_psicosociales_Red_de_automanejo_de_enfermedades_cronicas (accessed on 14 April 2024).
46. Lorig, K.; Stewart, A.; Ritter, P.; González, V.; Laurent, D.; Lynch, J. *Outcome Measures for Health Education and Other Health Care Interventions*, 1st ed.; no. 11; SAGE Publications: Thousand Oaks, CA, USA, 1996.
47. Gonzales, V.; Lorig, K.; Laurent, D.; Castagnola, L. *Taller Virtual Tomando Control de su Salud. Manual para Líderes*; Self-Management Resource Center: Palo Alto, CA, USA, 2021.
48. Reglamento de la Ley General de Salud en Materia de Investigación para la Salud. México. 2014. Available online: https://www.diputados.gob.mx/LeyesBiblio/regley/Reg_LGS_MIS.pdf (accessed on 5 August 2024).
49. Asociación Médica Mundial Declaración de Helsinki de la AMM—Principios Éticos para las Investigaciones Médicas en seres Humanos. Available online: https://www.wma.net/es/policies-post/declaracion-de-helsinki-de-la-amm-principios-eticos-para-las-investigaciones-medicas-en-seres-humanos/ (accessed on 9 June 2024).
50. Puccinelli, P.J.; da Costa, T.S.; Seffrin, A.; de Lira, C.A.B.; Vancini, R.L.; Nikolaidis, P.T.; Knechtle, B.; Rosemann, T.; Hill, L.; Andrade, M.S. Correction to: Reduced level of physical activity during COVID-19 pandemic is associated with depression and anxiety levels: An internet-based survey. *BMC Public Health* **2021**, *21*, 613. [CrossRef] [PubMed]

Disclaimer/Publisher's Note: The statements, opinions and data contained in all publications are solely those of the individual author(s) and contributor(s) and not of MDPI and/or the editor(s). MDPI and/or the editor(s) disclaim responsibility for any injury to people or property resulting from any ideas, methods, instructions or products referred to in the content.

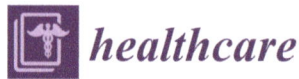

Article

The Value of the COVID-19 Yorkshire Rehabilitation Scale in the Assessment of Post-COVID among Residents of Long-Term Care Facilities

Łukasz Goździewicz [1,*], Sławomir Tobis [2], Michał Chojnicki [3,4], Katarzyna Wieczorowska-Tobis [1,5] and Agnieszka Neumann-Podczaska [1]

[1] Geriatric Unit, Department of Palliative Medicine, Poznań University of Medical Sciences, 61-245 Poznań, Poland
[2] Department of Occupational Therapy, Poznań University of Medical Sciences, 60-781 Poznań, Poland
[3] Department of Immunobiology, Poznań University of Medical Sciences, 60-806 Poznań, Poland
[4] Department of Infectious Diseases, Józef Struś Hospital, 61-285 Poznań, Poland
[5] Department of Human Nutrition and Dietetics, Poznań University of Life Sciences, 60-624 Poznań, Poland
* Correspondence: lukasz.gozdziewicz@gmail.com

Abstract: The COVID-19 Yorkshire Rehabilitation Scale (C19-YRS) is a patient-reported outcome measure designed to assess the long-term effects of COVID-19. The scale was validated and is commonly used in the general population. In this study, we assess the utility of the C19-YRS in evaluating the post-COVID burden among residents of long-term care facilities with a mean age of 79. C19-YRS and Barthel index evaluations were performed among 144 residents of long-term care facilities reporting new or worsened symptoms or functioning three months after convalescence from COVID-19. The C19-YRS-based screening showed that 70.9% of COVID-19 convalescents had ≥ 1 complaint three months after recovery. The highest C19-YRS-scored symptoms (indicating a higher burden) were breathlessness, fatigue, and cognitive and continence problems; however, symptomatology was very heterogeneous, revealing a high complexity of the disease in older persons. The mean total C19-YRS score was higher in hospitalized patients (n = 78) than in the outpatient group (n = 66) ($p = 0.02$). The functioning subscale of the C19-YRS strongly correlated with the Barthel index, with r = −0.8001 ($p < 0.0001$). A moderately strong correlation existed between retrospectively reported C19-YRS-based functioning and the Barthel index score reported before illness (r = 0.7783, $p < 0.0001$). The C19-YRS is instrumental in evaluating the consequences of COVID-19 among long-term-care residents. The assessment allows for a broad understanding of rehabilitation needs.

Keywords: COVID-19 Yorkshire Rehabilitation Scale; long-term care; post-COVID-19

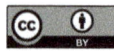

1. Introduction

Older people, or those with immunodeficiencies and/or chronic diseases, remain at high risk of severe COVID-19, even in a time of the dominance of SARS-CoV-2 Omicron sublineages with less virulence compared to those present at the beginning of the pandemic [1]. Institutional long-term care, i.e., nursing homes and social assistance facilities, are places in which all these factors cumulate, making the community of residents, older people living with advanced physical and/or cognitive disabilities, one of the populations most vulnerable to COVID-19. Long-term care facilities became hotspots for COVID-19 spread and mortality due to increased transmission rates [2–4]. While SARS-CoV-2 Omicron sublineages are unlikely to cause an excess of severe COVID-19 similar to that of the SARS-CoV-2 Delta variant, hospital admissions and deaths are still frequent, i.e., reported in about 4–5% of residents [5]. Subsequent outbreaks of COVID-19 in long-term care facilities may sustain strain on residents, personnel, and the healthcare system [6,7]. However, while populational vaccinations decreased the risk of the severe clinical course of COVID-19, they were insufficient to prevent infection outbreaks in long-term care facilities [7,8].

The COVID-19 burden does not end with convalescence. Health deficits may persist for months after the illness and substantially impact patients' functioning. Post-COVID, also called long-COVID or post-acute sequelae of SARS-CoV-2 infection, was included in the ICD-10 classification in September 2020 and is defined by the World Health Organization as a condition that occurs in individuals with a history of probable or confirmed SARS-CoV-2 infection, usually three months from the onset of COVID-19, with symptoms that last for at least two months. Symptoms, which most commonly include but are not limited to fatigue, shortness of breath, and cognitive dysfunction, cannot be explained by an alternative diagnosis [9]. The literature lists over 200 different symptoms [9,10]; however, no minimal number of symptoms is required for diagnosis at present [9]. Attempts to develop a new post-COVID definition revealed that the algorithm needs to incorporate the symptoms and characteristics of patients, e.g., sex, age, and comorbidities [11]. Patients living in long-term facilities are an example of a population in need of determining the burden of post-COVID and guiding care and rehabilitation programs.

It is well established that the functioning of COVID-19 convalescents living in long-term care facilities, assessed by the standard activities of daily living (ADL) questionnaire, is impaired months after the illness [12,13]. Assessment tools like the Barthel index, which is frequently used as an administrative evaluation of patients in nursing and social assistance homes, capture functioning without quantifying the whole dimension of post-COVID syndrome. This may limit the perception of the healthcare needs of patients. A comparison of the COVID-19 Yorkshire Rehabilitation Scale (C19-YRS) with the EuroQoL 5D-5L, a health-related quality of life assessment tool, showed higher symptom detection with a disease-specific scale and agreement in shared items [14]. Proper tools that allow for the screening of post-COVID syndrome are needed for tailored interventions in patients with post-COVID. Patients of an advanced age and with multimorbidity frequently report post-COVID symptoms, i.e., fatigue, pain, depression, and cognitive dysfunction. It is challenging to distinguish between post-COVID and other clinical entities. Minimally, the evaluation must include at least a comparison of possible syndrome manifestations with health and functioning before the illness. Retrospective assessment of pre-COVID-19 symptoms or functioning reported by patients can be biased.

The pandemic had a substantial impact on residents of long-term care institutions which is not only measured by the number of infections and deaths but also adverse effects on physical and emotional functioning [15–17]. Knowledge about post-COVID in older adults, especially those with the most advanced age, complex disabilities, and frailty, is scant [18]. This also concerns the population of residents of long-term facilities who experience rapid and significant functional decline following infection and disabilities persisting from a few to several months [12,13,19]. Investigating delayed COVID-19 effects on long-term care residents requires careful attention to their intricate health issues and varied physical, psychological, and social needs.

As mentioned before, the C19-YRS is a patient-reported outcome measure assessing the long-term effects of COVID-19. The scale encompasses 22 items divided into symptom severity, functional disability, and global health score and provides a comprehensive insight into the persisting symptoms of post-COVID. The clinical utility and psychometric attributes of the C19-YRS were appraised in an observational study of patients with post-COVID attending rehabilitation clinics (n = 187). The analysis employed classical psychometric methods, encompassing data quality, scaling assumptions, targeting, reliability, and validity assessments. The results indicated that the internal consistency was high, with good concordance between the overall perception of health and the patients' reports of symptoms, functioning, and disability [20]. After the study, the C19-YRS was largely adopted in clinical practice, and a modified version (C19-YRSm) was devised as a patient-reported outcome measure for post-COVID syndrome which has been validated for patient assessment and monitoring in this context [21,22]. In summary, the C19-YRS was studied in populations of individuals recovering from COVID-19, particularly those experiencing lingering symptoms. Through this scale, healthcare professionals can garner a more profound understanding of SARS-CoV-2's enduring impacts, aiding in enhancing rehabilitation approaches [23–26]. The C19-YRS had not yet been studied in a population of patients of the most advanced age. Frailty and functional dependency in older patients make them more susceptible to severe and critical conditions, often exhibiting complex and atypical symptoms in sequelae [27,28]. This necessitates a comprehensive approach to their assessment and care management. The C19-YRS captures a broad range of symptoms, functioning items, and overall health, has validated reliability, and focuses on patient-reported outcomes [20–22,29].

In this study, we assessed the utility of the C19-YRS to evaluate the post-COVID burden among residents of long-term care facilities. We correlated the total C19-YRS score with the Barthel index to assess the agreement between two measures: the COVID-19-specific and standard measures used in long-term care facilities. In addition, we assessed agreement between retrospectively assessed functioning and the Barthel index assessed before the illness, which is routinely and regularly evaluated in every patient in long-term care facilities in Poland.

2. Materials and Methods

2.1. Study Design

This was a cross-sectional study utilizing some historically reported data. The study was conducted in four social assistance facilities and one nursing home in Wielkopolska, Poland. SARS-CoV-2 infection was confirmed using PCR testing from nasopharyngeal swabs. All enrolled residents of long-term care facilities were COVID-19 convalescents who reported worsening (including the presence of new symptoms) health or/and functioning three months after their recovery from COVID-19. The screening for the worsening was performed using the C19-YSR. Collected characteristics included sex, age at the time of illness, and COVID-19 course, which was characterized as requiring hospitalization or not. A Barthel index assessment was conducted parallel to the C19-YRS assessment. All assessments were performed three months after recovery from COVID-19.

The C19-YRS questionnaire was obtained from Rory J. O'Connor, Leeds General Infirmary, Leeds, United Kingdom, and translated into Polish. The C19-YRS has four subscales: symptom severity (including the most common symptoms of post-COVID), functional disability, additional symptoms, and overall health. The severity of every symptom (breathlessness, cough, swallowing/nutrition, fatigue, continence, pain/discomfort, cognition, anxiety, depression, and post-traumatic stress disorder (PTSD)), five functional disabilities (communication, mobility, personal care, other ADL, and social role), additional symptoms (palpitations, dizziness/falls, weakness, sleep problems, fever, and skin rash), and overall health were evaluated at scale from 0 to 10 each, where 0 indicated no symptom/disability and 10 indicated extreme symptom severity/disability. Routinely, the C19-YRS includes item evaluation at assessment and before COVID-19, i.e., patients rated all symptoms, functioning, and overall health pre-COVID-19 and at the assessment. All patients reporting impairment in ≥ 1 item or an additional symptom were included in the analysis.

Patients or their legal representatives gave informed consent before data collection. This study was authorized by the Ethics Committee at the Poznan University of Medical Sciences (approval note KB-247/21).

2.2. Data Analysis and Interpretation

The total C19-YRS scores were calculated as the sum of all subscores (22 items). Data were analyzed descriptively, with continuous variables presented as means with SD values and as counts and percentages in the case of nominal variables. Symptom severity and functional impairment assessed by the C19-YRS were considered severe when the mean subscale sore was ≥ 6, moderate in the range from 3 to 5.9, and mild when <3 [29]. Continuous variables in subgroups of patients were compared using a one-way ANOVA. Pearson's correlation was used to analyze the association between the Barthel index and the total C19-YRS score or its functioning subscale. To assess agreement between C19-YRS-based functioning retrospectively reported by patients and functioning reported before COVID-19, we assessed the correlating retrospective assessment of functioning performed three months after the illness with the Barthel index score values assessed before COVID-19. Correlations were interpreted based on the method of Chan, Y.H., 2003 [30]. Values $p < 0.05$ were considered statistically significant. Statistical analysis was performed using MedCalc 22.013 statistical software (MedCalc Software, LLC, Ostend, Belgium). Data were visualized using MedCalc software or Microsoft Office Package.

3. Results

3.1. Patients

In total, 203 patients were screened for the presence of symptoms of worsening functioning or the presence of new symptom(s) three months after COVID-19. Among them, 144 patients (70.9%) declared during the C19-YRS-based screening at least one new complaint or worsening symptoms, functioning, or overall health compared to the period before COVID-19. Participant characteristics and two main analyzed measures are shown in Table 1. Patients aged ≥80 years comprised 52.1% and patients aged ≥65 years comprised 91.6% of the overall population. None of the patients were vaccinated against COVID-19.

Table 1. Patient characteristics.

Characteristic	Patients (n = 144)
Mean age, years (±SD)	78.7 (±9.4)
Males, n (%)	57 (39.6%)
Clinical course of COVID-19, n (%)	
Not hospitalized	66 (45.8%)
Requiring hospitalization	78 (54.2%)
Mean C19-YRS score (±SD)	51.2 (±31.2)
Mean Barthel index score (±SD)	57.1 (±33.5)

3.2. Post-COVID Burden Evaluated Using the COVID-19 Yorkshire Rehabilitation Scale

The mean (±SD) total C19-YRS score was 51.2 (±31.2) (Table 1). Women had a higher mean total C19-YRS score than men (57.1 ± 30.4 vs. 42.4 ± 30.4, $p = 0.005$). The total C19-YRS score was higher in hospitalized patients than those who remained in a long-term care facility during the illness (56.9 ± 31.4 vs. 44.7 ± 29.8, $p = 0.0190$); however, there was no difference between the mean Barthel index scores in groups of hospitalized and non-hospitalized patients (53.6 ± 33.5 vs. 61.3 ± 33.2, $p = 0.1750$).

Based on the mean C19-YRS symptom subscale, 3.5% of patients (n = 5) had severe symptoms, 16.7% had moderate symptoms (n = 24), and 79.9% had mild symptoms (n = 115). Severe functional impairment was present in 30.6% of patients (n = 44), moderate functional impairment was present in 31.9% (n = 46), and mild functional impairment was present in 37.5% (n = 54). Table 2 shows symptoms, functioning, overall health, and additional symptom subscores. The mean symptom and functional subscores were higher in the hospitalized patient group than in non-hospitalized patients (Table 2). These two groups had no difference in overall health and additional symptom subscales ($p = 0.9$).

The symptoms with the highest severity in the overall population were breathlessness, fatigue, cognition disturbances, and continence (Table 2 and Figure 1a). The most affected functioning areas were other ADLs, social roles, and personal care (Table 2 and Figure 1c). Among other symptoms, the highest severity was reported for weakness, sleep problems, and dizziness/falls (Table 2). Symptoms that were more severe in the hospitalized than in the non-hospitalized group were breathlessness, continence, depression, and PTSD (Table 2 and Figure 1b). Patients who were hospitalized due to COVID-19 had a higher impairment of mobility, personal care, and communication than patients who spent the illness in a social assistance facility or nursing home (Table 2 and Figure 1d). There was no difference in overall health perception between hospitalized and not-hospitalized groups, and the only additional symptom that was more severe in the non-hospitalized group than in the hospitalized group was skin rash (Table 2).

Table 2. The COVID-19 Yorkshire Rehabilitation Scale symptom, functioning, overall health, and additional symptom items analyzed in all patients and subgroups of non-hospitalized and hospitalized patients. Higher scores indicate higher symptom severity or greater impairment of functioning.

C19-YRS Subscales/Items, Mean ± SD	All Patients	Non-Hospitalized Patients	Hospitalized Patients	p-Value *
Symptom subscale	18.6 ± 17.4	14.9 ± 15.9	21.7 ± 18.2	0.0180
Breathlessness	2.7 ± 3.2	1.6 ± 2.4	3.7 ± 3.5	<0.001
Cough	1.0 ± 2.2	1.2 ± 2.4	0.8 ± 2.0	0.2170
Swallowing/nutrition	1.0 ± 2.5	0.8 ± 2.3	1.1 ± 2.7	0.6270
Fatigue	2.6 ± 3.1	2.6 ± 3.1	2.7 ± 3.1	0.8630
Continence	2.4 ± 3.7	1.6 ± 3.2	3.1 ± 4.0	0.0150
Pain/discomfort	1.8 ± 2.9	1.7 ± 2.7	1.8 ± 3.0	0.7530
Cognition	2.5 ± 3.4	2.0 ± 3.0	2.9 ± 3.7	0.1470
Anxiety	1.7 ± 2.9	1.3 ± 2.6	2.0 ± 3.0	0.1310
Depression	1.9 ± 2.7	1.4 ± 2.5	2.3 ± 2.8	0.0410
PTSD [1]	1.1 ± 2.4	0.6 ± 1.7	1.4 ± 2.8	0.0320
Functioning subscale	21.5 ± 14.8	18.6 ± 14.4	24.0 ± 17.2	0.0280
Communication	2.0 ± 3.1	1.3 ± 2.6	2.5 ± 3.4	0.0200
Mobility	4.3 ± 3.7	3.4 ± 3.5	5.1 ± 3.7	0.0070
Personal care	4.8 ± 3.7	4.0 ± 3.7	5.5 ± 3.6	0.0150
Other ADL	5.4 ± 3.8	5.1 ± 4.0	5.8 ± 3.6	0.2620
Social role	4.9 ± 4.2	4.8 ± 4.3	5.1 ± 4.3	0.6290
Health overall	5.3 ± 2.5	5.3 ± 2.3	5.3 ± 2.7	0.9630
Additional symptom subscale	5.9 ± 7.6	5.8 ± 7.6	5.9 ± 7.8	0.9440
Palpitations	0.7 ± 1.8	0.8 ± 1.8	0.7 ± 1.8	0.7970
Dizziness/falls	1.3 ± 2.1	1.1 ± 1.9	1.4 ± 2.3	0.3840
Weakness	2.0 ± 2.4	1.8 ± 2.0	2.3 ± 2.7	0.2310
Sleep problems	1.4 ± 2.4	1.5 ± 2.6	1.3 ± 2.3	0.6430
Fever	0.2 ± 0.7	0.2 ± 0.7	0.1 ± 0.7	0.6400
Skin rash	0.3 ± 1.3	0.6 ± 1.8	0.1 ± 0.4	0.0100

* one-way ANOVA for comparison between non-hospitalized and hospitalized groups. ADL, activities of daily living; [1] PTSD, post-traumatic stress disorder; SD, standard deviation.

3.3. Correlation between Assessment Tools

The total C19-YRS score was fairly correlated with the Barthel index, with r = −0.4749 (95% CI: −0.5925 to −0.3376) (p < 0.0001) (Figure 2a). There was a very strong correlation between the sum of the functioning scores of the C19-YRS and the Barthel index with r = −0.8001 (95% CI: −0.8521 to −0.7324) (p < 0.0001) (Figure 2b). Finally, to assess agreement between patients reporting functioning status which, with the C19-YRS, is reported at assessment and retrospectively for before COVID-19, we correlated these answers with the Barthel index scores recorded before infection as part of routine assessment. There was a moderately strong correlation between the retrospectively reported functioning subscale of the C19-YRS and the historic Barthel index, with r = −0.7783 (95% CI: −0.8359 to −0.7038) (p < 0.0001).

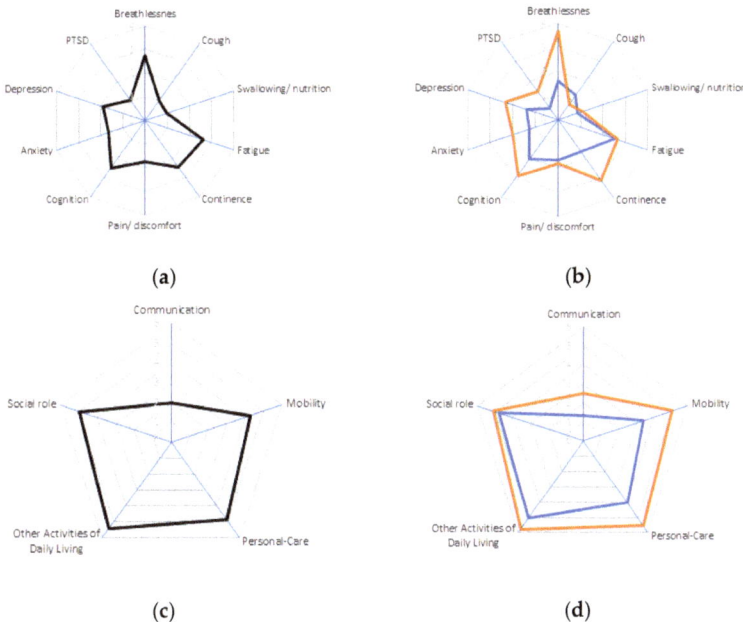

Figure 1. The mean COVID-19 Yorkshire Rehabilitation Scale item scores. Symptom scores overall (**a**) and in subgroups of patients (**b**) hospitalized due to COVID-19 (red) or with a course of the disease not requiring hospitalization (blue). Functioning scores overall (**c**) and in subgroups of patients (**d**) hospitalized due to COVID-19 (red) or with a course of the disease not requiring hospitalization (blue). Higher scores indicate higher symptom severity or highgreater impairment of functioning. The range of scores was from 0 to 10. PTSD, post-traumatic stress disorder.

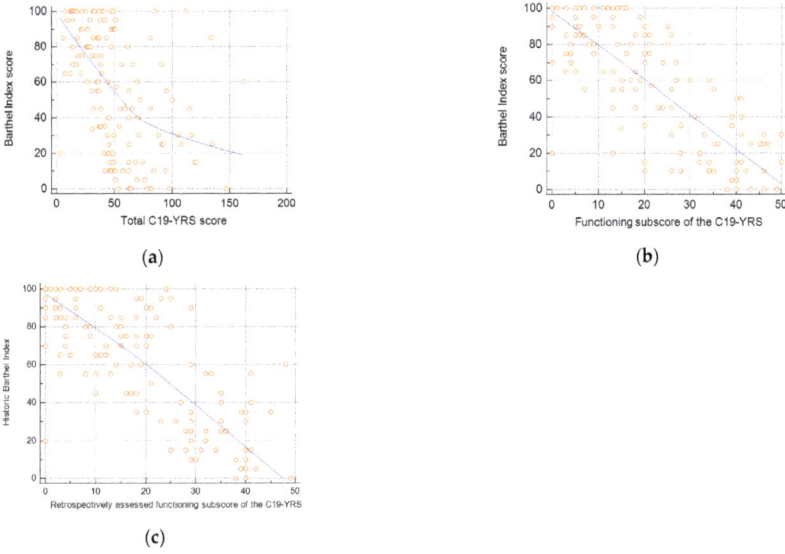

Figure 2. Correlation between total C19-YRS score and the Barthel index (**a**), functioning subscale of the C19-YRS and the Barthel Index (**b**), and retrospective assessment of functioning subscale of the C19-YRS and historic Barthel index assessed before SARS-CoV-2 infection (**c**).

4. Discussion

We are in a time of intensified research on post-COVID syndrome; however, data available for older adults are scant [31–33]. Here, we screened for post-COVID symptoms and impaired ADLs in the group of COVID-19 convalescents living in long-term care facilities. About half of the patients reporting new symptoms or worsening of functioning were over 80 years old. These patients are rarely included in studies assessing the post-COVID burden [18].

Functioning is one of the primarily impaired aspects of post-COVID sequelae and was extensively studied before in a population of residents of long-term facilities [12,13,19]. Older patients more frequently reported mobility and ADL impairments [23]. The current results confirm that the highest scores, indicative of impairment, were attributed to different functioning items compared to symptom items. Almost every third patient had severe functional impairment, highlighting the need for rehabilitation. Similar to the earlier observations of Zhang et al., 2023 [24], the female sex was associated with the presence of post-COVID symptoms.

A fair correlation existed between the total C19-YRS score and the Barthel index, but a robust agreement existed between the functioning subscore and ADL measure. This indicates that the C19-YRS itself captures a broad view of post-COVID-associated dysfunction. This may result in more positive screening results, as shown previously [14]. The use of the C19-YRS for screening post-COVID symptoms in the group of patients ≥ 55 years old resulted in 81.2% of patients reporting ≥ 1 symptom. The COVID-19-specific measure allowed for broader symptom detection than other measures. Interestingly, in our study, the standard ADL measure used in long-term care facilities did not capture the difference in functioning between hospitalized and non-hospitalized patients, while the C19-YRS did. Both symptoms and functional impairment were more pronounced in patients who required a hospital stay due to COVID-19. Patients who needed hospital admission demanded more health resources after the acute infection [26].

In our study, severe symptoms were reported by only a few patients, unlike the previous study [29]. For the first time, we used the C19-YRS to screen a population of advanced-age persons, whereas earlier, general practitioners referred adult patients (men age 47) to a multidisciplinary rehabilitation service [29]. These differences largely contribute to our cohort's lower severity of symptoms compared to earlier experiences with the C19-YRS. The sampling method largely affects the subscales values recorded, e.g., the random sampling of patients (mean age 67) without severe cognitive and functional impairments, based only on the history of COVID-19 but not the presence of worsening symptoms, functioning, or overall health resulted in lower scores than those reported here [34]. The questionnaire allows one to capture a heterogeneous spectrum of symptoms. In line with earlier reports about the post-COVID manifestation in older adults, fatigue and dyspnea were the most prevalent [24,33]. In our study, breathlessness was the most severe among patients hospitalized due to COVID-19, whereas fatigue severity was similar to that of non-hospitalized patients. Respiratory failure during COVID-19 requiring hospitalization correlated with respiratory symptoms in the year after acute SARS-CoV-2 infection [35]. Breathlessness-associated hypoxia, in combination with long-term care immobilization and social isolation, may result in cardiovascular and neurological complications [36]. Timely respiratory rehabilitation intervention may improve the prognosis. Respiratory rehabilitation benefits pulmonary function, quality of life, and anxiety in older persons with COVID-19 [37]. Another important finding is a relatively high incontinence severity in the studied group. Awareness about the association between SARS-CoV-2 infection and this symptom is low, leading to inadequate early management. The underlying mechanism is poorly understood and possibly involves a low-grade bladder infection, autonomic nervous system dysfunction, pudendal nerve neuropathy, and weakened musculoskeletal systems impacting pelvic floor function [38,39]. It should be stressed that continence (and also swallowing, fever, and skin rash) were infrequently reported in the C19-YRS validation study, and their contribution to the overall measurement properties of the scale was limited [20]. In our study, incontinence was the fourth most severe symptom, indicating that the assessment may have more value in older age than in middle-aged adults. The only symptom more severe in non-hospitalized patients than hospitalized patients was a skin rash; however, the severity was low. Since post-COVID is thought to be an immune disorder driven by viral persistence, molecular mimicry, and other pathological mechanisms [40], a worsening or new-onset disease, autoimmune condition, or allergic reaction is frequently described in the literature [41,42]. The risk of autoimmune manifestation increased over time since the onset of infection and was independent of the patient's demographics. The main factor predicting the risk of manifestation was COVID-19 in an outpatient setting [42]. The authors considered that anti-inflammatory treatment during hospital stays may decrease the autoimmune burden of post-COVID. The exact mechanism may protect hospitalized patients from developing a skin rash.

We found a very strong correlation between self-reported functioning and ADL evaluated independently. The Barthel index and ADL score are the most frequently used assessments to evaluate the functional impact of COVID-19 across different contexts [43]. However, there are differences between the functioning subscales of the C19-YRS and the Barthel index, e.g., C19-YRS covers communication and social role, which is missing in the Barthel index [20,44]; there was a very strong correlation between both assessments. The severity of symptoms reported by patients can be biased to some degree by subjectivity in their evaluation and a general perception of the worsening of care associated with practices and policies related to the pandemic. In addition to the correlation of assessments performed simultaneously, the functioning reported by patients in the pre-COVID time strongly correlated with the Barthel index score. This indicates that using the C19-YRS gives reliable results regarding functioning before and after the illness and that recall bias is limited, at least with respect to ADL. The reliability of the retrospective assessment, especially in patients for whom syndrome symptoms may overlap with other comorbidities, was one of the issues requiring investigation [18].

This study had limitations. It was a cross-sectional study that captured the long-term COVID-specific burden three months after recovery from the disease; however, post-COVID is not a stable phenomenon, and symptoms and functioning may fluctuate over time, which was evidenced in the nursing home resident population [16]. The study design limited conclusions about the scale's sensitivity to change. Due to its cross-sectional nature, this study did not allow for a confirmation of the diagnosis of post-COVID since symptoms should persist for at least two months [9]. It is important to note that the mean scores recorded in different studies largely depend on the sampling method. This study was conducted in the early phase of the pandemic, before the populational availability of vaccines. Receiving a primary vaccination and additional doses was associated with fewer post-COVID symptoms in an older population [24]. This and the evolution of SARS-CoV-2 sublineages need to be considered when interpreting data from cohorts from different times. Advanced-age patients are often frail and have physical limitations, cognitive impairments, and dementia, which could affect their ability to accurately report symptoms using the C19-YRS, as well as exacerbate post-COVID symptoms. This and low digital literacy in the population limits the use of the remote version of the scale [45] since many patients would require assistance in answering questions. The symptoms of comorbidities might overlap with post-COVID symptoms, making it challenging to attribute specific symptoms to the syndrome impact accurately.

5. Conclusions

The C19-YRS is instrumental in evaluating the consequences of COVID-19 among long-term care residents. The original version of the measure can be used in populations of patients of an advanced age, or at least incontinence should be assessed due to its high severity in this group. The assessment allows for a broader understanding of post-COVID needs compared to the sole activities of daily living check. Information about symptoms and functioning may guide proper rehabilitation interventions since targeting symptoms has been shown to impact functioning. The C19-YRS pre-COVID-19 assessment of functioning had very good agreement with a baseline ADL assessment, confirming the measure's reliability in assessing status before the illness.

Author Contributions: Conceptualization, Ł.G., A.N.-P. and K.W.-T.; methodology, Ł.G., A.N.-P. and K.W.-T.; validation, Ł.G., A.N.-P., M.C. and S.T.; formal analysis, Ł.G., A.N.-P. and S.T.; investigation, Ł.G. and A.N.-P.; resources, Ł.G. and A.N.-P.; writing—original draft preparation, Ł.G. and A.N.-P.; writing—review and editing Ł.G., M.C., A.N.-P., K.W.-T. and S.T.; visualization M.C., Ł.G. and A.N.-P.; supervision, A.N.-P.; project administration, A.N.-P.; funding acquisition, A.N.-P. All authors have read and agreed to the published version of the manuscript.

Funding: This research received no external funding.

Institutional Review Board Statement: The study was approved by the Ethics Committee of the Poznan University of Medical Sciences (approval note KB-247/21, 10 March 2021).

Informed Consent Statement: Informed consent was obtained from all subjects involved in the study or their legal representatives.

Data Availability Statement: The data supporting this study's findings are available from the corresponding author upon reasonable request.

Acknowledgments: Marcin Balcerzak of Medink provided medical writing services.

Conflicts of Interest: The authors declare no conflict of interest.

References

1. World Health Organization. *Therapeutics and COVID-19. Living guideline, 10 November 2023*; World Health Organization: Geneva, Switzerland, 2023.
2. Burki, T. England and Wales see 20,000 excess deaths in care homes. *Lancet* **2020**, *395*, 1602. [CrossRef] [PubMed]
3. Quigley, D.D.; Dick, A.; Agarwal, M.; Jones, K.M.; Mody, L.; Stone, P.W. COVID-19 Preparedness in Nursing Homes in the Midst of the Pandemic. *J. Am. Geriatr. Soc.* **2020**, *68*, 1164–1166. [CrossRef]
4. Szczerbińska, K. Could we have done better with COVID-19 in nursing homes? *Eur. Geriatr. Med.* **2020**, *11*, 639–643. [CrossRef]
5. Krutikov, M.; Stirrup, O.; Nacer-Laidi, H.; Azmi, B.; Fuller, C.; Tut, G.; Palmer, T.; Shrotri, M.; Irwin-Singer, A.; Baynton, V.; et al. Outcomes of SARS-CoV-2 omicron infection in residents of long-term care facilities in England (VIVALDI): A prospective, cohort study. *Lancet Healthy Longev.* **2022**, *3*, e347–e355. [CrossRef] [PubMed]
6. Wilson, W.W.; Keaton, A.A.; Ochoa, L.G.; Hatfield, K.M.; Gable, P.; Walblay, K.A.; Teran, R.A.; Shea, M.; Khan, U.; Stringer, G.; et al. Outbreaks of SARS-CoV-2 Infections in Nursing Homes during Periods of Delta and Omicron Predominance, United States, July 2021–March 2022. *Emerg. Infect. Dis.* **2023**, *29*, 761–770. [CrossRef] [PubMed]
7. Reeve, L.; Tessier, E.; Trindall, A.; Aziz, N.; Andrews, N.; Futschik, M.; Rayner, J.; Didier'Serre, A.; Hams, R.; Groves, N.; et al. High attack rate in a large care home outbreak of SARS-CoV-2 BA.2.86, East of England, August 2023. *Eurosurveillance* **2023**, *28*, 2300489. [CrossRef]
8. Danis, K.; Fonteneau, L.; Georges, S.; Daniau, C.; Bernard-Stoecklin, S.; Domegan, L.; O'Donnell, J.; Hauge, S.H.; Dequeker, S.; Vandael, E.; et al. High impact of COVID-19 in long-term care facilities, suggestion for monitoring in the EU/EEA, May 2020. *Eurosurveillance* **2020**, *25*, 2000956. [CrossRef]
9. Soriano, J.B.; Murthy, S.; Marshall, J.C.; Relan, P.; Diaz, J.V. A clinical case definition of post-COVID-19 condition by a Delphi consensus. *Lancet Infect. Dis.* **2022**, *22*, e102–e107. [CrossRef]
10. Davis, H.E.; Assaf, G.S.; McCorkell, L.; Wei, H.; Low, R.J.; Re'em, Y.; Redfield, S.; Austin, J.P.; Akrami, A. Characterizing long COVID in an international cohort: 7 Months of symptoms and their impact. *eClinicalMedicine* **2021**, *38*, 101019. [CrossRef]
11. Thaweethai, T.; Jolley, S.E.; Karlson, E.W.; Levitan, E.B.; Levy, B.; McComsey, G.A.; McCorkell, L.; Nadkarni, G.N.; Parthasarathy, S.; Singh, U.; et al. Development of a Definition of Postacute Sequelae of SARS-CoV-2 Infection. *JAMA* **2023**, *329*, 1934–1946. [CrossRef]
12. Trevissón-Redondo, B.; López-López, D.; Pérez-Boal, E.; Marqués-Sánchez, P.; Liébana-Presa, C.; Navarro-Flores, E.; Jiménez-Fernández, R.; Corral-Liria, I.; Losa-Iglesias, M.; Becerro-de-Bengoa-Vallejo, R. Use of the Barthel Index to Assess Activities of Daily Living before and after SARS-COVID 19 Infection of Institutionalized Nursing Home Patients. *Int. J. Environ. Res. Public Health* **2021**, *18*, 7258. [CrossRef]
13. Goździewicz, Ł.; Tobis, S.; Chojnicki, M.; Chudek, J.; Wieczorowska-Tobis, K.; Idasiak-Piechocka, I.; Merks, P.; Religioni, U.; Neumann-Podczaska, A. Long-Term Impairment in Activities of Daily Living Following COVID-19 in Residents of Long-Term Care Facilities. *Med. Sci. Monit.* **2023**, *29*, e941197. [CrossRef]
14. Ayuso García, B.; Romay Lema, E.; Rabuñal Rey, R. Useful tools in post-COVID syndrome evaluation. *Med. Clin.* **2022**, *159*, e33–e34. [CrossRef]

15. Levere, M.; Rowan, P.; Wysocki, A. The Adverse Effects of the COVID-19 Pandemic on Nursing Home Resident Well-Being. *J. Am. Med. Dir. Assoc.* **2021**, *22*, 948–954.e2. [CrossRef] [PubMed]
16. Carnahan, J.L.; Lieb, K.M.; Albert, L.; Wagle, K.; Kaehr, E.; Unroe, K.T. COVID-19 disease trajectories among nursing home residents. *J. Am. Geriatr. Soc.* **2021**, *69*, 2412–2418. [CrossRef] [PubMed]
17. Greco, G.I.; Noale, M.; Trevisan, C.; Zatti, G.; Dalla Pozza, M.; Lazzarin, M.; Haxhiaj, L.; Ramon, R.; Imoscopi, A.; Bellon, S.; et al. Increase in Frailty in Nursing Home Survivors of Coronavirus Disease 2019: Comparison With Noninfected Residents. *J. Am. Med. Dir. Assoc.* **2021**, *22*, 943–947.e3. [CrossRef] [PubMed]
18. Sorensen, J.M.; Crooks, V.A.; Freeman, S.; Carroll, S.; Davison, K.M.; MacPhee, M.; Berndt, A.; Walls, J.; Mithani, A. A call to action to enhance understanding of long COVID in long-term care home residents. *J. Am. Geriatr. Soc.* **2022**, *70*, 1943–1945. [CrossRef] [PubMed]
19. Clark, S.E.; Bautista, L.; Neeb, K.; Montoya, A.; Gibson, K.E.; Mantey, J.; Kabeto, M.; Min, L.; Mody, L. Post-acute sequelae of SARS-CoV-2 (PASC) in nursing home residents: A retrospective cohort study. *J. Am. Geriatr. Soc.* **2023**. [CrossRef] [PubMed]
20. O'Connor, R.J.; Preston, N.; Parkin, A.; Makower, S.; Ross, D.; Gee, J.; Halpin, S.J.; Horton, M.; Sivan, M. The COVID-19 Yorkshire Rehabilitation Scale (C19-YRS): Application and psychometric analysis in a post-COVID-19 syndrome cohort. *J. Med. Virol.* **2022**, *94*, 1027–1034. [CrossRef] [PubMed]
21. Sivan, M.; Halpin, S.; Gee, J.; Makower, S.; Parkin, A.; Ross, D.; Horton, M.; O'Connor, R. The self-report version and digital format of the COVID-19 Yorkshire Rehabilitation Scale (C19YRS) for Long COVID or Post-COVID syndrome assessment and monitoring. *ACNR* **2021**, *20*, 16–19. [CrossRef]
22. Sivan, M.; Preston, N.; Parkin, A.; Makower, S.; Gee, J.; Ross, D.; Tarrant, R.; Davison, J.; Halpin, S.; O'Connor, R.J.; et al. The modified COVID-19 Yorkshire Rehabilitation Scale (C19-YRSm) patient-reported outcome measure for Long Covid or Post-COVID-19 syndrome. *J. Med. Virol.* **2022**, *94*, 4253–4264. [CrossRef] [PubMed]
23. Mińko, A.; Turoń-Skrzypińska, A.; Rył, A.; Tomska, N.; Bereda, Z.; Rotter, I. Searching for Factors Influencing the Severity of the Symptoms of Long COVID. *Int. J. Environ. Res. Public Health* **2022**, *19*, 8013. [CrossRef] [PubMed]
24. Zhang, D.; Chung, V.C.; Chan, D.C.; Xu, Z.; Zhou, W.; Tam, K.W.; Lee, R.C.; Sit, R.W.; Mercer, S.W.; Wong, S.Y. Determinants of post-COVID-19 symptoms among adults aged 55 or above with chronic conditions in primary care: Data from a prospective cohort in Hong Kong. *Front. Public Health* **2023**, *11*, 1138147. [CrossRef]
25. Ho, F.F.; Xu, S.; Kwong, T.M.H.; Li, A.S.; Ha, E.H.; Hua, H.; Liong, C.; Leung, K.C.; Leung, T.H.; Lin, Z.; et al. Prevalence, Patterns, and Clinical Severity of Long COVID among Chinese Medicine Telemedicine Service Users: Preliminary Results from a Cross-Sectional Study. *Int. J. Environ. Res. Public Health* **2023**, *20*, 1827. [CrossRef]
26. Ayuso García, B.; Besteiro Balado, Y.; Pérez López, A.; Romay Lema, E.; Marchán-López, Á.; Rodríguez Álvarez, A.; García País, M.J.; Corredoira Sánchez, J.; Rabuñal Rey, R. Assessment of Post-COVID Symptoms Using the C19-YRS Tool in a Cohort of Patients from the First Pandemic Wave in Northwestern Spain. *Telemed. J. E Health* **2023**, *29*, 278–283. [CrossRef]
27. Guo, T.; Shen, Q.; Guo, W.; He, W.; Li, J.; Zhang, Y.; Wang, Y.; Zhou, Z.; Deng, D.; Ouyang, X.; et al. Clinical Characteristics of Elderly Patients with COVID-19 in Hunan Province, China: A Multicenter, Retrospective Study. *Gerontology* **2020**, *66*, 467–475. [CrossRef] [PubMed]
28. Bull-Otterson, L.; Baca, S.; Saydah, S.; Boehmer, T.; Adjei, S.; Gray, S.; Harris, A. Post–COVID Conditions Among Adult COVID-19 Survivors Aged 18–64 and ≥65 Years—United States, March 2020–November 2021. *MMWR Morb. Mortal Wkly. Rep.* **2022**, *71*, 713–717. [CrossRef]
29. Sivan, M.; Parkin, A.; Makower, S.; Greenwood, D.C. Post-COVID syndrome symptoms, functional disability, and clinical severity phenotypes in hospitalized and nonhospitalized individuals: A cross-sectional evaluation from a community COVID rehabilitation service. *J. Med. Virol.* **2022**, *94*, 1419–1427. [CrossRef]
30. Chan, Y.H. Biostatistics 104: Correlational analysis. *Singap. Med. J.* **2003**, *44*, 614–619.
31. Cohen, K.; Ren, S.; Heath, K.; Dasmariñas, M.C.; Jubilo, K.G.; Guo, Y.; Lipsitch, M.; Daugherty, S.E. Risk of persistent and new clinical sequelae among adults aged 65 years and older during the post-acute phase of SARS-CoV-2 infection: Retrospective cohort study. *BMJ* **2022**, *376*, e068414. [CrossRef]
32. Wan, E.Y.F.; Zhang, R.; Mathur, S.; Yan, V.K.C.; Lai, F.T.T.; Chui, C.S.L.; Li, X.; Wong, C.K.H.; Chan, E.W.Y.; Lau, C.S.; et al. Post-acute sequelae of COVID-19 in older persons: Multi-organ complications and mortality. *J. Travel. Med.* **2023**, *30*, taad082. [CrossRef]
33. Daitch, V.; Yelin, D.; Awwad, M.; Guaraldi, G.; Milić, J.; Mussini, C.; Falcone, M.; Tiseo, G.; Carrozzi, L.; Pistelli, F.; et al. Characteristics of long-COVID among older adults: A cross-sectional study. *Int. J. Infect. Dis.* **2022**, *125*, 287–293. [CrossRef] [PubMed]
34. Tamadoni, N.; Bakhtiari, A.; Nikbakht, H.A. Psychometric properties of the COVID-19 Yorkshire Rehabilitation Scale: Post-COVID-19 syndrome in Iranian elderly population. *BMC Infect. Dis.* **2024**, *24*, 77. [CrossRef] [PubMed]
35. Steinbeis, F.; Thibeault, C.; Doellinger, F.; Ring, R.M.; Mittermaier, M.; Ruwwe-Glösenkamp, C.; Alius, F.; Knape, P.; Meyer, H.J.; Lippert, L.J.; et al. Severity of respiratory failure and computed chest tomography in acute COVID-19 correlates with pulmonary function and respiratory symptoms after infection with SARS-CoV-2: An observational longitudinal study over 12 months. *Respir. Med.* **2022**, *191*, 106709. [CrossRef] [PubMed]
36. Poloni, T.E.; Medici, V.; Zito, A.; Carlos, A.F. The long-COVID-19 in older adults: Facts and conjectures. *Neural Regen. Res.* **2022**, *17*, 2679–2681. [CrossRef] [PubMed]

37. Liu, K.; Zhang, W.; Yang, Y.; Zhang, J.; Li, Y.; Chen, Y. Respiratory rehabilitation in elderly patients with COVID-19: A randomized controlled study. *Complement. Ther. Clin. Pract.* **2020**, *39*, 101166. [CrossRef] [PubMed]
38. Emordi, V.; Lo, A.; Bisharat, M.; Malakounides, G. COVID-19-Induced Bladder and Bowel Incontinence: A Hidden Morbidity? *Clin. Pediatr.* **2024**, *63*, 10–13. [CrossRef] [PubMed]
39. Farooq, M.; Faisal, S.; Rashid, H.H.; Sharif, K.; Habib, H.; Khalid, M.; Hassan, Z. Frequency of Urinary Incontinence Among Post COVID Males. *J. Health Rehabil. Res.* **2023**, *3*, 174–180. [CrossRef]
40. Dotan, A.; Muller, S.; Kanduc, D.; David, P.; Halpert, G.; Shoenfeld, Y. The SARS-CoV-2 as an instrumental trigger of autoimmunity. *Autoimmun. Rev.* **2021**, *20*, 102792. [CrossRef]
41. Marín, J.S.; Mazenett-Granados, E.A.; Salazar-Uribe, J.C.; Sarmiento, M.; Suárez, J.F.; Rojas, M.; Munera, M.; Pérez, R.; Morales, C.; Dominguez, J.I.; et al. Increased incidence of rheumatoid arthritis after COVID-19. *Autoimmun. Rev.* **2023**, *22*, 103409. [CrossRef]
42. Chang, R.; Yen-Ting Chen, T.; Wang, S.I.; Hung, Y.M.; Chen, H.Y.; Wei, C.J. Risk of autoimmune diseases in patients with COVID-19: A retrospective cohort study. *eClinicalMedicine* **2023**, *56*, 101783. [CrossRef]
43. Pizarro-Pennarolli, C.; Sánchez-Rojas, C.; Torres-Castro, R.; Vera-Uribe, R.; Sanchez-Ramirez, D.C.; Vasconcello-Castillo, L.; Solís-Navarro, L.; Rivera-Lillo, G. Assessment of activities of daily living in patients post COVID-19: A systematic review. *PeerJ* **2021**, *9*, e11026. [CrossRef] [PubMed]
44. Wade, D.T.; Collin, C. The Barthel ADL Index: A standard measure of physical disability? *Int. Disabil. Stud.* **1988**, *10*, 64–67. [CrossRef] [PubMed]
45. Sivan, M.; Rocha Lawrence, R.; O'Brien, P. Digital Patient Reported Outcome Measures Platform for Post-COVID-19 Condition and Other Long-Term Conditions: User-Centered Development and Technical Description. *JMIR Hum. Factors* **2023**, *10*, e48632. [CrossRef] [PubMed]

Disclaimer/Publisher's Note: The statements, opinions and data contained in all publications are solely those of the individual author(s) and contributor(s) and not of MDPI and/or the editor(s). MDPI and/or the editor(s) disclaim responsibility for any injury to people or property resulting from any ideas, methods, instructions or products referred to in the content.

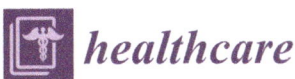

Review

Horticultural Therapy for Individuals Coping with Dementia: Practice Recommendations Informed by Related Non-Pharmacological Interventions

Matthew J. Wichrowski [1,*] and Monica Moscovici [2]

[1] Rusk Rehabilitation, NYU Grossman School of Medicine, NYU Langone Health, New York, NY 10016, USA
[2] NYU Langone Health, New York, NY 10016, USA; monica.moscovici@nyulangone.org
* Correspondence: matthew.wichrowski@nyulangone.org

Abstract: Dementia care currently presents a challenge to healthcare providers on many levels. The rapid increase in the number of people with dementia and the costs of care certainly contribute to these challenges. However, managing the behavioral and psychological symptoms of dementia (BPSDs) has become one of the most significant tasks in providing care and can lead to poor health and well-being outcomes, not only for the people living with dementia (PLWD) but also for those providing their care. Cost-effective, easily implemented, highly adaptable, empirically based alternatives are needed. Interventions such as Horticultural Therapy (HT), which is naturally informed by Montessori-Based Methods for Dementia and sensory reminiscence therapies, meets these qualifying factors. This article, based on a review of current best practices and clinical experience, hopes to provide recommendations for such an intervention along with special considerations for PLWD and adaptations for different acuity levels. With additional safe and effective, person-centered, non-pharmacological interventions available for the complex cognitive and neuropsychiatric manifestations of this disease, a better care milieu can be provided, improving the quality of life for both patients and caregivers. This article also identifies the need for continued research into the synergistic effects of person-centered behavioral and psychosocial interventions combined with environmental approaches to provide the optimal healing environment for those coping with dementia.

Keywords: nature-based therapy; horticultural therapy; complementary therapies; dementia care; Montessori methods

1. Introduction

Currently, more than 55 million people are living with dementia (PLWD) worldwide, and almost 10 million new cases are being diagnosed every year. The global economic cost of dementia reached 1.3 trillion (US dollars) in 2019, trickling down to healthcare facilities and personal costs [1]. Considering these numbers as well as the American baby boomer population, set to begin aging into the dementia range, [2,3], the amount of PLWD (and their ensuing costs) is predicted to triple by 2050 [4]. This exponential rise in elderly individuals with dementia will require an equal increase in more specialized care. Memory care facilities can achieve such care by integrating newer, cost-effective, non-pharmacological, and person-centered alternatives to managing the complex and increasing cases of dementia [2].

Dementia is a general term that encompasses the "loss of memory and other mental abilities severe enough to interfere with daily life" [5]. Such losses are brought on by physical changes in the brain due to a multitude of causes ranging from diseases such as alcoholism and Huntington's disease to traumatic brain injuries and family genetics. Although Alzheimer's is the most common type of dementia, there are four other major categories of dementia. These include Vascular Dementia, Frontal-Temporal Dementia, Lewy Body/Parkinson's Dementia, and Mixed-Type Dementia. Over 120 causes, variations, and types of dementia have been identified thus far [5]. Even though they can all be defined by the decline in cognitive function, people living with all types of dementia also "experience a host of neuropsychiatric symptoms" [6]. Although most often studied in patients with Alzheimer's disease, the resulting behavioral and psychological symptoms of dementia (BPSD) can complicate any cause of dementia. These symptoms are among the most distressing to both patients with dementia and their caregivers. They are also associated with a high economic burden [7]. Such symptomatology can also become an underlying cause of common adverse outcomes for PLWD. These possible outcomes can include "increased hospitalization, decreased quality of life, and increased distress among patients and caregivers, as well as being associated with more rapid progression of disease" [6,8]. This article aims to address two BPSDs that can be especially difficult for daily caregivers. Agitation and depression affect emotional, social, and ultimately physical domains. They are also the symptoms that are most proven to be alleviated by Horticultural Therapy [8].

The neuropsychological symptoms of depression and agitation tend to cause social isolation and/or low self-worth with a lack of motivation. This amalgamation of symptoms and their affected domains causes a highly decreased quality of life. Not only does this affect the person with the disease but also their family, friends, and caretakers [6].

Caretaker well-being is an important consideration in this equation. Formal caregiver training and ability has been proven to be the most effective BPSD intervention [9]. Trained caregivers are more likely to provide "high-intensity care" and handle behavioral problems. They also report higher amounts of strain, mental and physical health problems, and caregiver burnout [10]. The psychological well-being of a dementia caregiver can also affect their care recipient. This often stems from the negative aspects of caregiving which in turn increases the chances of depression and anxiety in their care recipient [11]. The CDC estimates that about 60% of dementia caregivers suffer from high rates of emotional distress and approximately 40% report symptoms of depression [12].

Considering these factors, the alleviation of BPSDs becomes highly important for PLWD and their immediate circle, especially caretakers, affecting the level of care they can provide [13,14]. Identifying effective neuropsychiatric symptom management techniques in PLWD, benefiting both patient and caregiver well-being, has become an important clinical goal. To that end, this article aims to offer helpful information for staff, caretakers, and activity providers.

Using non-pharmacological means can provide both physical and emotional symptom alleviation [15]. These interventions are often preferred due to the possibility of medications precipitating neurobehavioral disturbances [6,16]. Proven alternatives that help with BPSDs include Montessori-Based Practices, the agency of choice/motor independence, and sensory reminiscence therapy [16–32]. These practices and their benefits naturally inform the provision of Horticultural Therapy (HT). HT is defined as the use of gardening activities for therapeutic exercise aimed at meeting individual treatment goals [33]. Studies from a systematic review utilizing HT and sensory gardens in caring for patients with dementia showed significant improvements in agitation levels as well as time spent engaged in activity. These results show encouraging possibilities for administrators in care facilities to use HT in caring for patients with dementia [4]. Utilizing such interventions can provide a clinically relevant, person-centered approach to meet the needs of increasing populations of persons coping with dementia and their caretakers.

2. Aim

The aim of this article is to explore contributions from the field of horticultural therapy as informed by associated non-pharmacological approaches to explore current aspects of dementia care, and in particular, to offer design and practice recommendations specifically tailored to the needs and clinical goals of those coping with dementia in its various forms.

A search and analysis of both the relevant classical and current literature was performed. With this, in combination with clinical expertise, the authors hope to integrate findings to offer safe, cost-effective, person-centered intervention options for BPSD management in patients and additionally reducing caretaker burden.

3. Methods: Data Sources and Search Strategies

Google Scholar and Pub Med were searched with the keywords: 'sensory gardens and dementia' (6650 results), 'gardens and dementia' (17,000 results), 'dementia and behavioral challenges' (17,000 results) and 'horticultural therapy and dementia' (3020 results). Articles were assessed for a date range of 'since 2020'. Articles were reviewed and discussed by authors. Criteria for selection included meta-analysis, review articles, RCTs, quantitative studies having high 'n' and utilizing validated scales, and mixed-method studies with high 'n' and validated scales. Consideration of earlier studies included foundational works and "classic studies". Further citations were derived from mining the reference lists from previous articles. Lastly, articles addressing unique approaches and interventions were explored for additional unique contributions to patient care according to the aims of the paper. Utilizing open-access journal articles was a key consideration in the literature search to enable wider ease of access. The large number of results precluded a systematic review, so the above-mentioned criteria combined with clinical expertise and author discussion guided the reference selections. Fifty-nine articles were chosen to inform the recommendations in this article.

4. Results: Evaluating Practices Supporting Person-Centered BPSD Management

The management of BPSDs is a highly individualized process. Following a thorough assessment by appropriate medical professionals, it is important to address any possible contributing medical problems or medication effects [9]. Concerns regarding the use of pharmacological therapies are addressed. In addition, non-pharmacological approaches shown to impact behavioral symptoms in dementia care are explored.

4.1. Pharmacological Therapy

Patients with dementia often are prescribed multiple medications. While pharmaceuticals that address medical problems and pain associated with dementia are important in managing BPSDs, there is evidence that some of these medications may be contributing to BPSDs. The reduction or discontinuation of medications associated with increases in BPSDs, as approved by medical personnel, could significantly improve BPSDs and associated difficulties [9]. For example, a recent study showed that "reducing anticholinergic burden by at least 20% significantly reduced the severity and frequency of BPSD and decreased caregiver burden" [34]. Drug–drug interactions should also be considered when reviewing or making changes to medications.

While psychiatric medications can help ease BPSDs, side effects can be just as problematic as the symptoms they are designed to combat [35,36]. While polypharmacy increases the possibility of negative side effects, it may even cause more serious issues "such as falls, strokes, or death" [6,36]. Due to such issues, pharmacological interventions should only be prescribed when "behaviors pose a significant safety risk" or if the person coping with dementia is extremely distressed. Although there is a lack of strong clinical evidence concerning the research and implementation of non-pharmacological interventions, the lack of adverse effects makes them promising options for managing BPSDs in situations that are not imminently dangerous. These interventions should include patients as well as their formal caregivers for best outcomes [9].

4.2. Horticultural Therapy

E.O. Wilson's Biophilia hypothesis states there is an innate biological and evolutionary connection between humans and nature [37] which has significant effects on mood. The findings of a recent meta-analysis indicate "that exposure to natural environments had a medium to large effect on both increasing positive affect and decreasing negative affect" [38].

It has been shown that human beings have a natural fascination and attraction to certain qualities of nature.

Another important foundational theory in HT work is Attention Restoration Theory (ART). When environments contain the features of being away, fascination, compatibility, and extent, it allows for effortless attention to nature that can offer rest and restoration from mental fatigue [39]. The ability to pay attention to one's environment and focus on one's goals is an important function in life. HT has the potential to impact many domains of function and can provide mental, physical, cognitive, emotional, social, and spiritual benefits.

The American Horticultural Therapy Association (AHTA) defines HT as an activity-based process that is part of a predetermined treatment plan in which "the process itself is considered the therapeutic activity rather than the end product". This type of nature-based therapy can be utilized as part of a stand-alone or team treatment approach. Therapeutic Horticulture (TH) is a closely aligned practice that aims to improve well-being through active or passive involvement with nature. TH uses the "restorative value of nature to provide an environment conducive to mental repose, stress-reduction, emotional recovery, and the enhancement of mental and physical energy". A TH session focuses on the psychological, physical, and social needs of its participants [33].

These activities (HT and TH) can be easily implemented in a variety of settings. Interventions can range from adjusting and enhancing an already existing garden (specializing its features to meet the needs of the particular populations it serves while adding biophilic features) to hands-on indoor planting or sensory-based herbal craft activities. These activities can further be graded to reflect the ability level of the participants and provide an appropriate level of challenge to assist in meeting their clinical goals. Specific areas in physical, emotional, cognitive, and social domains can be targeted [40].

Although a relatively new field, HT can provide benefits for a wide range of different populations. This can include, but is not limited to, veterans; people with special needs, psychiatric disorders, and experience of substance abuse; those in skilled nursing and assisted living settings, cancer (both active and remission) patients; those in hospices/palliative care; and homeless populations [33]. HT can also be immensely relevant to PLWD. Cognitively, the use of HT/TH has been proven to stimulate memory [41] and improve attention capacity [42]. Guided horticultural activities can also serve to exercise sequencing abilities, generalizable to Activities of Daily Living (ADLs). Psychologically, it has been shown to improve mood [43] as well as quality of life [44], while alleviating depression [45]. HT/TH can improve personal worth [46], increase self-esteem [47], and enable a sense of pride and accomplishment. Lastly, it has even been shown to provide an increased sense of stability [48].

The above benefits are incredibly useful to PLWD and offer great possibilities for the improvement of BPSDs. In fact, the effects of sensory gardens and HT programs on improvements in agitation levels and time spent engaged in activity are well documented for PLWD. Not only is engagement shown to increase but the overall time spent in inactivity is shown to decrease when HT or sensory gardens are introduced. Even personal affect became more positive during HT when compared to traditional activities [4]. Planting and other nature-based activities, whether inside or outside, can promote a range of benefits, including the provision of a non-threatening, mood-enhancing activity that promotes social opportunity, inclusion, and support.

4.3. Montessori Method for Dementia

HT is naturally informed by the Montessori Method for treating dementia, which has been developing for the past twenty years and is used on an international scale. Multiple reviews have reported that Montessori-Based Practices (MBPs) improved constructive engagement and had positive affects [16–18], as well as improved eating behaviors and cognition [14]. The method typically involves "(a) identifying an activity of interest that is reflective of the individual's skill level; (b) making use of familiar materials and objects;

(c) breaking the activity down into small steps; and (d) inviting the individual to complete the task themselves" [18]. This process can increase the meaningfulness of the activity and improve motivation and participation.

The Montessori Method relies heavily on the agency of choice and motor independence, another proven alternative to the use of pharmaceuticals to help treat BPSDs. "As human beings... we need to be proud of our abilities and feel respected by other people. These experiences can often be hard to achieve for persons with dementia, partly due to symptoms of dementia and also due to other persons' reactions" [19]. This often results in feelings of "failure/weakness, losing face, ignorance, and conflict" [20]. Therefore, a feeling of agency and independence becomes very important.

However, because PLWD can have inaccurate perceptions of their abilities, it is practical to provide both the opportunity to use their abilities while also getting help to remember how they previously used these abilities [19]. The solution to this balance between independence and support/safety is to do things together—as in doing things with the person rather than for them, focusing on the things the person can do, rather than the things they cannot—while offering reassurance, encouragement, and plenty of time and patience, if needed [21].

It is important for the participant to be involved as much as possible in each step of the activity, with the focus being on maximizing individual contributions during the process rather than on the product. This can simply mean enabling a person to do things their way, within reason [22], while also offering a potent tool for therapeutic improvement. A comparison of behaviors and speech, both before and after utilizing this method, showed that PLWD displayed a decrease in the negative themes that come with perceived inability and its BPSDs, as well as an actual increase in ability [23].

4.4. Sensory and Reminiscence Therapy

Sensory stimulation refers to a variety of techniques and activities used to exercise the senses, helping to increase alertness and reduce agitation [24]. It includes visual, olfactory, tactile, gustatory, auditory, and even kinesthetic stimulation [25]. Offering the opportunity to explore stimuli can bring a state of pleasant relaxation [26]. The addition of nature-based stimuli has the potential to further increase the benefits. Studies show that "simply touching wood or viewing an image of roses for just three minutes can induce beneficial physiological responses" including relaxation and stress reduction [49]. Because nature allows for effortless attention and connection [37,39], it offers easily attainable benefits with less work for both patient and caregiver.

The beneficial effects of sensory stimulation can extend beyond relaxation (both physical and mental) to opportunities for returning to a sense of self. According to some dementia literature, "cognitive impairment in people with dementia is often regarded as representing a loss of self-hood" [19,29]. This view implies the separation of the mind from the body. The significance of embodiment for PLWD (and all people in general) cannot be stressed enough [27]. People living with dementia tend to dissociate from their mind, body, and current moment in time [19]. The grounding action of embodiment not only helps release stress and improve mental well-being [28] but can offer some reprieve from symptoms of dementia [24]. Sensory stimulation therapy offers the opportunity to reorient to the present by producing increased mental alertness through sensory stimulation. At the same time, it has the potential to improve quality of care by expanding on the caretakers' communication methods for connecting with patients suffering from BPSDs [29]. Therapeutic benefits can be enhanced through the addition of reminiscence therapy, which typically ties to the sense of smell but can also include the other senses and even muscle memory.

For over 50 years, memory stimulation in the form of reminiscence therapy has been seen to help process life events and prepare for death, with added benefits of mental and psychosocial well-being [30,31]. Knowledge and understanding of a patient's personal history and preferences can contribute significantly to optimal patient care and patient satisfaction [30]. Both knowledge of history, through the eyes of the patient, along with information gained from sensory stimulation allows caretakers to view patients as individuals and find new meaning in their behaviors that push past just being symptoms of a disease and more towards a way of relating, especially if there is an unmet need [29]. Reminiscence, life review, cognitive stimulation, music therapy, and aromatherapy, among others, have demonstrated positive effects on people living with dementia [32] and their caretakers [29]. While these therapies were in use, such as music played during baths, multisensory stimulation room sessions, and aromatherapy or massage, BPSDs were greatly improved. Communication, quality of life, and function also improved [27]. As a result of such improvements, the staff members experienced equal improvement, with a sense of excitement that made them even more willing to implement such interventions [29].

5. Variations of Horticultural Therapy Implementation

5.1. Doing and Being in the Garden

There are a multitude of ways in which HT can be implemented, depending on team treatment goals, contraindications, acuity level, and participant preference. When implementing HT, whether indoors or in a specially designed garden, it is helpful to consider both passive benefits as well as specific prescribed activity as a therapeutic exercise designed to meet the clinical needs or treatment goals of participants. The combination of setting and activity creates the potential for a wide range of therapeutic benefits for an equally wide range of abilities [6].

5.2. Memory Gardens—Setting Up for Being in the Garden

Memory Gardens can be a great therapeutic horticulture option. To be effective, they should contain several elements while avoiding elements possibly hazardous to people with dementia (Table 1).

Table 1. Recommended garden elements and their precautions [50–52].

Element	Considerations	Precautions
Boundary	<ul><li>An enclosed space is important for safety</li><li>It is equally important for visitors not to feel confined so screening fences and walls with hanging plants can minimize feelings of being closed in.</li></ul>	<ul><li>Using locks on all gate apparatuses or openings in between fences is important since PLWD may be able to open regular gates and divisions in fences that are not meant to be opened</li></ul>
Walkway	<ul><li>A paved path with a contrasting color on each side/edge to help delineate safe, flat walking areas from uneven garden/planted areas should be provided</li><li>This path should be wide, solid, and safe enough to support wheelchair access</li><li>The path should form a loop that begins and ends in the same location, with focal points that provide interest along the way and signs that clearly mark an extra wide entry/exit and other important points</li><li>Interpretive signage can add cognitive stimulation and provide a sense of meaning to enhance the garden experience</li></ul>	<ul><li>Raised curbs or edges along walkways can cause a tripping hazard</li><li>Walkways that are not level are discouraged for similar fall risk issues</li></ul>
Planting Considerations	<ul><li>Plants that engage all of the senses offer many opportunities for stimulation including:<ul><li>fuzzy and/or textured plants;</li><li>fragrant plants;</li><li>edible plants (i.e., mint and other culinary herbs).</li></ul></li><li>Plants that are most likely to be familiar to garden visitors such as geraniums and roses</li><li>Something of interest for every season (i.e., a mix of annuals and different perennials)</li></ul>	<ul><li>Plants with any kind of toxicity level are discouraged</li><li>Plants with thorns, spikes, or sharp edges, like cacti, lemongrass, certain roses, and bromeliads are discouraged</li><li>Plants that have a chance of causing contact dermatitis are discouraged</li><li>Plants whose pollen causes common allergic reactions (i.e., chamomile is in the ragweed family and may cause a reaction for people allergic to ragweed pollen) are discouraged</li></ul>

Having a garden that allows visitors to be able to orient themselves through visual cues and a path that brings them back to where they started provides increased feelings of control, self-confidence, and reinforcement to go outdoors [46]. The ability to go outdoors, especially alone (when assessed by a clinician or caregiver based on current weather conditions and the affect/ability of the individual), has been shown to alleviate the agitation and depression symptoms of dementia [53]. Just being around plants can help enhance that effect, offering a soothing, quieting quality [6,48,54]. Providing a space for gathering, sheltered from the sun, can offer opportunities for socialization, another characteristic that can improve such symptoms [50–52]. This mix of structured and unstructured activity is a key benefit to garden visitors as they can be afforded the autonomy to move about as they see fit while providing a degree of direction. The garden setting can also provide a purposeful way to meet ambulatory goals. A well-designed garden enhances enjoyment, increases utilization, and creates a rich setting to employ HT activities that further enhance the therapeutic potential for participants. This effective combination magnifies the overall experience of horticultural therapy [6].

Including one or two sturdy garden beds that PLWD can sit, stand, or pull their wheelchair up to can be a great feature for annual plantings such as herbs, geraniums, or other familiar flowers. Most people tend to have some past personal experience with or memory of gardening, especially with parents or grandparents. This is great for stimulating reminiscence. The fragrant olfactory stimulation offered by herbs is also recommended in any memory garden. Benches (facing the path) and railings, at appropriate intervals, are also recommended to allow garden visitors to rest or gain a little extra help while still feeling independent [50–52]. If no easily reachable outdoor space is available, an enclosed balcony or sunroom with a garden bed that PLWD can stand, sit, or bring their wheelchair up to can also achieve similar benefits. The use of low-cost LED lighting can embellish existing light in a darker space and create a warm-feeling, plant-friendly space for participants to enjoy, especially in winter when conditions outside may not be conducive for garden visits. Settings with hot summers will also benefit from a climate-controlled indoor garden.

5.3. Planting Activity Example—Setting Up for Doing in (and out of) the Garden

The addition of prescribed garden activities aimed at meeting the clinical and personal goals of the individual adds a range of benefits for participants. Being able to learn about and explore a few plants (usually no more than three depending on cognitive status) offers cognitive stimulation and the opportunity to reminisce and engage with texture, thickness, and different color variations while smelling and feeling the soil or the plant itself. This provides the opportunity to exercise most of the senses. Choosing one's plant also provides some personal control and choice during the activity and an increased sense of meaning.

The simple act of transplanting a starter plant into a larger pot, to give it more room to grow, offers metaphorical opportunities for discussion which can positively impact self-confidence and motivation [32,46–48]. This can also be expanded to propagation and seed starting activities as well, for extra variety, keeping in mind that simple steps, adapted for different acuity levels (Table 2), done one at a time, while offering two or three choices for each step tend to work well.

Such activities set up the conditions for easy, sequential task completion, allowing opportunities for independent tiered goal achievement. Sequencing exercises performed during an enjoyable, structured task may generalize to other important tasks requiring sequencing such as ADL skills [40]. Allowing participants to have a hand in every single step, even if with assistance, elicits a feeling of accomplishment and pride (Table 3) [19,21,41].

Table 2. Recommended adaptations for acuity levels when working with soil [40,55].

Level of Acuity	Adaptation	Sequence of Steps
Higher functionality—ability to stand	• Use soil placed in a big, wide container/bucket with high sides placed on a table or surface where participants can stably stand and mix	1. Mist/spray soil with water; 2. Mix soil; 3. Mist/spray perlite with water; 4. Mix perlite; 5. Then, mix perlite into soil (participants are usually good at choosing proper ratios on their own so have them decide what looks right); 6. Fill the empty pot one-third with soil; 7. Squeeze the pot with the plant inside to release roots; 8. Turn the pot upside down while holding the top of the soil between flat open fingers falling in between the plant; 9. Release the plant and place it right-side up into its new pot; 10. Fill all the empty spaces around the plant with soil.
Higher functionality—wheelchair	• Use soil placed in a container with lower sides so participants who are sitting down can see inside	
Medium functionality	• Use soil placed in a closed Ziplock bag for easier accessibility than in containers and more opportunity for finger mobility practice when mixing/squeezing with bare hands • This is an especially good option for patients who are reluctant to touch the soil or get their hands dirty	
Medium functionality—less tendency to eat materials	• Use measuring cups to add different amounts of perlite to the soil or to scoop the soil into pots • This can add some level of familiarity, especially if the participant was not a gardener	
Lower functionality and/or tendency to eat materials	• Use soil and perlite in closed Ziplock bags only • Move all materials away from the participant after completing each step • Work in a team or assembly line fashion	1. Keep the soil in a Ziplock bag and in the hands of an activity provider at all times; 2. Present the opened bag to allow one participant to mist the soil; 3. Close the Ziplock bag and have the next participant mix the soil in the closed bag; 4. With the Ziplock bag open in the hands of an activity provider, have one or two people take turns filling the new pot under supervision; 5. Allow the next participant to squeeze the pot with the plant inside to loosen its roots; 6. Have another participant turn the plant, along with its pot, upside down to release the plant from its pot and "tickle" its roots to spread them out a bit; 7. Have one participant make a hole in the pot from step 4 that is big enough for the plant and place the plant in the pot; 8. Allow the next participant to fill in the soil around the plant and pat it down to "tuck in the plant" and stabilize the roots.
For all Acuity Levels	• All equipment and materials used (e.g., trowels, plastic soil containers, bags and bins, water sprayer handles, pouches, seeds and seed containers/shakers, etc.) should be larger in size than normal for ease of use in this population and to prevent client frustration and feelings of helplessness while participating in the activity.	

Table 3. Recommendations for types of acuity-based assistance [40,55].

Level of Function	Assistance Strategy for Activity Providers/Caregivers
High	• Use mostly verbal cues with minimal physical assistance

Medium	• Ask the participant to do part of the task
	• For example:
	  ○ Hold the pot while you fill it with soil or vice versa;
	  ○ Hold dried herbs in an open hand while you use one hand to rub them or hold them in a flat open hand while you direct and tip them into the pouch;
	  ○ Hold and pull one side of the string or ribbon when making a knot to close the pouch.

Low	• Hand over hand, where your hands are over theirs, makes the activity easier
	• Or having the participant's hand over yours, squeezing when they want you to:
	  ○ Cut (with a scissor while pruning);
	  ○ Squeeze (the pot you are holding to loosen the roots);
	  ○ Write a letter on a plant label;
	  ○ Push the label into a predetermined spot.

Low functionality	• Total hand-over-hand physical assistance • Or demonstration while participant chooses options by where their gaze lands

Having something to take care of something (i.e., the finished plant project)—in a situation where people have little control over anything and others are doing everything for them—offers a feeling of control and usefulness in the world [44,46]. Not only does this bring cognitive, emotional, and psychosocial benefits, but it also enables the use of gross and fine motor skills. If there are standing tolerance goals, the planting activity can also be done in conjunction with other rehabilitation therapies.

5.4. Soil-Less Activity Example for Immunological Concerns

Planting and soil activities may not be appropriate for everyone. For example, some individuals prefer not to have any interaction with soil, even if wearing gloves. In some such cases, planting activities may become counterintuitive to the alleviation of agitation. There may also be situations in which soil is contraindicated due to specific immunological and infection concerns. These considerations and preferences should be assessed and evaluated by the medical team and activity staff, respectively.

While planting offers many opportunities for sensory practice, other activities such as an herbal aromatherapy sleep pouch activity can provide additional opportunities to exercise the senses while experiencing nature. Such activities can start with an exploration of different dried herbs while learning about their benefits. Next comes comparing their colors and shapes while feeling their textures and squeezing the herbs between a participant's palms or fingers. Listening to the noise they make when rubbed, and finally, smelling their released essential oils while reminiscing about memories can provide a powerful sensory experience [56].

Providing information about the benefits of the herbs, plus information about their historic uses at the start of the activity, offers cognitive and auditory stimulation. Offering three different herbs that are known to help with different parts of sleep [57,58] (like lavender, lemon balm, and rosemary) allows for the agency of choice, providing participants the option of refusing to use or interact with specific plant materials. Some people have very good reactions to certain smells, while others have negative reactions to the same smell. Exercising such preference in the agency of choice can be easily built into the activity.

This activity also offers an opportunity for the use of fine motor skills by squeezing and rubbing the herbs to release their essential oils (scent). Mixing and pouring the herbal blend into the pouch also offers gross motor stimulation, and so does ripping up tissues to fill the pouch and help distribute the herbs more evenly. Finally, squeezing and mixing the pouch once closed, to further distribute the materials inside and release their scent, allows for the use of fine finger motions. Completing such a project and putting it in between their pillow and pillow case can bring participants a sense of accomplishment and some ownership over their well-being. Lastly, this activity is not limited to immunocompromised participants alone. It can be used for the general dementia care population and can be adjusted to a spice blend sachet or herbal tea blend, with proper participant, nutritional, and safety considerations, by using a paper coffee filter and 6-inch cotton string, instead of a pre-made muslin or cotton pouch.

6. Special Considerations for People Living with Dementia

6.1. Memory Gardens—Being in the Garden

Montessori Methods for Dementia are known for focusing not only on supporting the individual but also on using and adapting the environment to provide safe yet independent engagement. The environment itself can be used as the support to promote independence. "We are unable to change the devastating effects of dementia but we can incorporate strategies and alter the environment while providing meaning and purpose to the day—so that the person not only engages in life, but has the opportunity to maintain, and even restore function" [22]. Memory gardens are the perfect example of this. On average, more than 90% of residents stay inside their unit in a lying down or sitting position throughout the day [53]. Offering enticing, supportive, and restoring environments can offer important interventions for such common issues.

Norton, 2023, has provided robust support from multiple studies that show a range of positive findings for therapeutic garden interventions when applied to help the dementia population. The majority of these findings were related to an increase in overall quality of life but there were many other benefits in individuals receiving this therapy, including a "reduction in agitation, positive changes in behavior, physical and mental health benefits, alleviation of social isolation, and potential changes in cortisol levels" [2].

6.2. HT Activities—Doing in (and out of) the Garden

Through this author's experience of providing a variety of HT activities for PLWD, a few things have proven themselves to work well. It may seem redundant, but introducing oneself, while pointing to a nametag—so participants can see where to find your name—and connecting yourself to something—such as holding up a plant—at the beginning of every HT activity is highly beneficial. So is a short introduction of what is about to happen and why. People in later stages of dementia often forget why they are there. Starting an activity without any introduction can be jarring under such circumstances. Simple transitions allowing for extra cognitive preparation and an understanding of what is expected from them during the activity can help alleviate this type of common discomfort. This is an element that can be easily forgotten by activity facilitators, especially if there is a mixed group of participants in varying stages of dementia, but such extra transition and preparation opportunities can be useful to ensure successful activity outcomes (Table 4) [29].

Table 4. Recommended material considerations.

Material	Special Considerations
Soil	• Use OMRI-certified organic, indoor potting mix as the planting medium
Perlite	• Add perlite to lighten the soil mix due to general tendencies of overwatering (a little too dry is better than too wet)
Tools	• Use plastic hand trowels and rakes as opposed to metal or wood • Use safety scissors when scissors are a necessity • Keep track of all tools at all times, especially at the end of the session
Any other added craft material or plant decoration	• Use materials larger than 1 1/2" to lower the possibility of choking [55]

Aromatherapeutic Herbs	• Avoid:
	  ○ Common allergenic plants such as those in the ragweed family (chamomile, mugwort);
	  ○ Finely ground herbs such as marjoram;
	  ○ Things that make one sneeze, such as hot pepper or other spices [59];
	  ○ Ingestion of Lemon Balm for those on sedatives or hypothyroid medication [56].

Safety concerns include areas of mental, emotional, and sensory safety. Some participants tend to have sensitivities to lights, sounds, and temperature. Sunglasses, earplugs or strategic microphone speakers, blankets, seating charts, and lots of support, encouragement, and patience for participants' independence can all address such sensitivities and allow for safe and successful sessions on all fronts. Likewise, working effectively with alternative behaviors maximizes safety and comfort during the activity and success in achieving HT goals (Table 5).

Lastly, PLWD are not always oriented to the present reality, but we can live in a shared reality while working on an activity together. This offers a therapeutic calm and stability for the activity participants and can also offer an opportunity for the formation of trust and bonds between the participants and caretakers. Allowing participants to feel comfortable and safe by not contradicting their current reality builds trust and can offer opportunities to see flickers of their personality and history. This can help caretakers understand and adapt better to individual needs and proclivities, while helping various activities of daily living proceed smoothly and providing a more positive work and therapeutic environment [23,25,26].

Table 5. Recommendations for working with alternative behaviors.

Behavior	Recommendations for Activity Providers/Caregivers
Dismantling projects	• Take the project back after each step or move it away from the participant • Make it a team/assembly line project
Short attention span/always fidgeting or doing things that may be unhelpful to the activity or group	• Provide reading/picture material as it coincides with the project while explaining, demonstrating, or working with everyone else • Provide small coloring, word search, or other printed games while everyone else is engaged in listening but make sure the coloring page or game is simple so as not to take too much time, losing their activity participation
Eating activity materials	• Make it a team/assembly line project • Put whatever materials you can in Ziplock bags (i.e., soil) • Use additional craft or plant decoration materials larger than 1 1/2" to eliminate choking hazards
Yelling/inappropriate remarks	• This can sometimes mean there is an unmet need so asking caretakers who know the participant best can let you know if everything is ok • Sometimes replying with an appropriate acknowledgment or word of conversation can help • In some cases, when all else fails, not paying attention to the behavior may be the only option.
Disagreements between participants	• Ask care staff to help seat participants according to who they get along with best and place persons that often have disagreements farthest apart • De-escalating situations with jokes or a tactful redirect back to the activity
Refusing to participate while being present	• Sometimes "participants" like to watch and just being present and out of their room is enough to meet their goals • Asking the "participant" for simple opinions on materials or placement can encourage a type of activity engagement • Invite the "participant" to be your assistant for the activity or for set up/clean up

7. Conclusions

Dementia care is moving towards a more multi-disciplinary, person-centered approach. However, with the predicted exponential rise in the number of dementia populations, an equal rise in more specialized care will become necessary [2,4]. It will benefit healthcare providers to begin exploring new options for the management of behaviors that are cost-effective, easily implemented, highly adaptable, and empirically based. The use of HT, including specifically designed therapeutic gardens guided by Montessori-Based Practices fulfills these criteria. The design and activity recommendations offered provide opportunities to reduce BPSDs as well as improve physical, cognitive, emotional, and social function. Along with increased engagement and decreased inactivity studies in a systematic review of HT use in caring for patients with dementia, there were decreased scores on the Cohen-Mansfield Agitation Inventory (CMAI). Such evidence should encourage administrators across care facilities to include HT interventions in their care milieu. To summarize, HT is a suitable, stimulating, and productive activity for dementia care programs.

Given the growing use of complementary therapies for promoting well-being, there is a need to study new therapeutic approaches that are available in order to find ways to ensure a high quality of care. This will help define and disseminate best practices for current and future PLWD across care settings [27] to provide the highest quality of life possible for those coping with dementia. Further research should continue to explore the relative benefits of complementary practices in dementia care including interventions such as HT alone or informed by other accepted practices. Sometimes the right mix of setting, approach, and activity can combine to have a robust therapeutic impact on the quality of life of those impacted by dementia and those who provide care for them.

8. Limitations and Future Directions

Although informed by a thorough review of the literature concerning the topics addressed, this paper is not meant to be a systematic review. Criteria for the literature chosen was based on the level of evidence with preference given to recent meta-analyses, review articles, randomized control trials, and higher 'n' studies utilizing validated scales to provide background and support for practice recommendations.

There are implicit limitations in this approach as compared to more systematic explorations. Yet, considering the aims of this paper, a wide array of current and classic resources provided information to back the treatment practices recommended herein. The recommendations provided are also informed by the successful clinical practice and experience of the authors. While there are limitations associated with this approach, it provides a sound foundation for patient-centered dementia care, with implications for exploring combinations of both environmental and clinical approaches to address relevant challenges and provide optimal care for those coping with this condition. There is potential in utilizing horticultural therapy and therapeutic garden design approaches to explore the efficacy of various interventions and combinations of interventions to maximize quality of life.

This exploration offers promise in developing a research agenda to further assess the effects of nature-based interventions in dementia care. In particular, nature-based interventions are well suited to address behavioral challenges and other clinically relevant issues such as supporting mood and providing cognitive and social stimulation to impact quality of life for both patient and caregiver. Effective combinations of unique interventions with synergistic effects are worthy of exploration in an experimental context.

Author Contributions: Conceptualization: M.J.W. and M.M.; Supervision, M.J.W.; Writing—original draft, M.M.; Writing—review and editing, M.J.W. and M.M. All authors have read and agreed to the published version of the manuscript.

Funding: This research received no external funding.

Institutional Review Board Statement: Not applicable.

Informed Consent Statement: Not applicable.

Data Availability Statement: Not applicable.

Conflicts of Interest: The authors declare no conflict of interest.

References

1. World Health Organization. Available online: https://www.who.int/news-room/fact-sheets/detail/dementia (accessed on 30 October 2023).
2. Norton, S.E. Therapeutic Gardening and Its Effects on Depressive Symptoms in Dementia Care. Bachelor's Thesis, University of Central Florida, Orlando, FL, USA, 2023. Available online: https://stars.library.ucf.edu/honorstheses/1396 (accessed on 20 January 2024).
3. Population Reference Bureau. 2018 World Population Data Sheet: With a Special Focus on Changing Age Structures. Available online: https://www.prb.org/wp-content/uploads/2018/08/2018_World-Population-data-sheet.pdf (accessed on 30 October 2023).
4. Lu, L.C.; Lan, S.H.; Hsieh, Y.P.; Yen, Y.Y.; Chen, J.C.; Lan, S.J. Horticultural therapy in patients with dementia: A systematic review and meta-analysis. *Am. J. Alzheimer's Dis. Other Dement.* **2020**, *35*, 1533317519883498. [CrossRef] [PubMed]
5. Positive Approach to Care. Available online: https://teepasnow.com/wp-content/uploads/sites/9/2022/01/Major-Types-of-Dementia-1.pdf (accessed on 17 December 2023).
6. Cummings, J.; Ritter, A.; Rothenberg, K. Advances in management of neuropsychiatric syndromes in neurodegenerative diseases. *Curr. Psychiatry Rep.* **2019**, *21*, 79. [CrossRef]
7. Beeri, M.S.; Werner, P.; Davidson, M.; Noy, S. The cost of behavioral and psychological symptoms of dementia (BPSD) in community-dwelling Alzheimer's disease patients. *Int. J. Geriatr. Psychiatry* **2002**, *17*, 403–408. [CrossRef]
8. Wheldon, T.; Metzler-Sawin, E. Therapeutic Horticulture for Dementia: A Systematic Review. *J. Gerontol. Nurs.* **2023**, *49*, 49–52. [CrossRef] [PubMed]

9. Bessey, L.J.; Walaszek, A. Management of Behavioral and Psychological Symptoms of Dementia. *Curr. Psychiatry Rep.* **2019**, *21*, 66. [CrossRef] [PubMed]
10. Sörensen, S.; Conwell, Y. Issues in dementia caregiving: Effects on mental and physical health, intervention strategies, and research needs. *Am. J. Geriatr. Psychiatry* **2011**, *19*, 491–496. [CrossRef]
11. Hwang, Y.; Kim, J. Influence of caregivers' psychological well-being on the anxiety and depression of care recipients with dementia. *J. Geriatr. Nurs.* **2023**, *55*, 44–51. [CrossRef]
12. Centers for Disease Control and Prevention (CDC). Available online: https://cmp.optimizely.com/cloud/%E2%80%94 (accessed on 17 December 2023).
13. Stella, F.; Forlenza, O.; Laks, J.; de Andrade, L.; de Castilho Cação, J.; Govone, J.; de Medeiros, K.; Lykestos, C.G. Caregiver report versus clinician impression: Disagreements in rating neuropsychiatric symptoms in Alzheimer's disease patients: Caregiver versus clinician in rating patient symptoms. *Int. J. Geriatr. Psychiatry* **2015**, *30*, 1230–1237. [CrossRef] [PubMed]
14. Warren, A. Behavioral and Psychological Symptoms of Dementia as a Means of Communication: Considerations for Reducing Stigma and Promoting Person-Centered Care. *Front. Psychol.* **2022**, *13*, 875246. [CrossRef]
15. Tilly, J.; Reed, P. Evidence on Interventions to Improve Quality of Care for Residents with Dementia in Nursing and Assisted Living Facilities. 2004. Available online: http://www.alz.org/documents/national/dementiacarelitreview.pdf (accessed on 21 January 2024).
16. Sheppard, C.L.; McArthur, C.; Hitzig, S.L. A systematic review of Montessori-based activities for persons with dementia. *J. Am. Med. Dir. Assoc.* **2016**, *17*, 117–122. [CrossRef]
17. Sander, L.H.; Sheppard, C.L. Implementing montessori methods for dementia: A scoping review. *Gerontologist* **2017**, *57*, e94–e114. [CrossRef]
18. Malone, M.L.; Camp, C.J. Montessori-based dementia programming: Providing tools for engagement. *Dementia* **2007**, *6*, 150–157. [CrossRef]
19. Norberg, A. Sense of self among persons with advanced dementia. In *Alzheimer's Disease [Internet]*; Wisniewski, T., Ed.; Codon Publications: Brisbane, Australia, 2019; Chapter 13. [CrossRef]
20. McAdams, D.P.; Hoffman, B.J.; Mansfield, E.D.; Day, R. Themes of agency and communion in significant autobiographical scenes. *J. Personal.* **1996**, *64*, 339–377. [CrossRef]
21. Alzheimer's Society 2022, Understanding and Supporting a Person with Alzheimer's. Available online: https://www.alzheimers.org.uk/get-support/help-dementia-care/understanding-supporting-person-dementia (accessed on 24 September 2023).
22. Association Montessori Internationale 2023 Montessori for Dementia, Disability and Aging. Available online: https://montessoridementia.org/sites/default/files/files/ChangingtheWorld.pdf (accessed on 22 September 2023).
23. Kihlgren, M.; Kuremyr, D.; Norberg, A.; Bråne, G.; Engström, B.; Karlsson, I.; Melin, E. Nurse-patient interaction after training in integrity promoting care at a long-term ward. Analysis of video-recorded morning care sessions. *Int. J. Nurs. Stud.* **1993**, *30*, 1–13. [CrossRef] [PubMed]
24. Gammeltoft, B.C. *Skjulte Handicaps hos Personer Ramt af Hjerneskade [Invisible Handicaps among Persons Suffering from Brain Injury]*; Forlaget FCT, Eligius: Høng, Denmark, 2005.
25. Vozzella, S. Sensory stimulation in dementia care: Why it is important and how to implement it. *Top. Geriatr. Rehabil.* **2007**, *23*, 102–113. [CrossRef]
26. Baker, R.; Bell, S.; Baker, E.; Gibson, S. A randomized controlled trial of the effect of multi-sensory stimulation (MSS) for people with dementia. *Br. J. Clin. Psychol.* **2001**, *40*, 81–96. [CrossRef] [PubMed]
27. Mileski, M.; Baar Topinka, J.; Brooks, M.; Lonidier, C.; Linker, K.; Vander Veen, K. Sensory and memory stimulation as a means to care for individuals with dementia in long-term care facilities. *Clin. Interv. Aging* **2018**, *13*, 967–974. [CrossRef] [PubMed]
28. Higgins, J. Understanding Selfhood to Elucidate the Phenomenology of Mindfulness. *Philosophia* **2022**, *50*, 551–566. [CrossRef]
29. Lykkeslet, E.; Gjengedal, E.; Skrondal, T.; Storjord, M.B. Sensory stimulation—A way of creating mutual relations in dementia care. *Int. J. Qual. Stud. Health Well-Being* **2014**, *8*, 23888. [CrossRef]
30. Lape, J. Using a multisensory environment to decrease negative behaviors in clients with dementia. *O.T. Prac.* **2009**, *14*, 9–13.
31. Tamura-Lis, W. Reminiscing—A tool for excellent elder care and improved quality of life. *Urol. Nurs.* **2017**, *37*, 142–151. [CrossRef]
32. Westerhof, G.J.; Bohlmeijer, E.T. Celebrating fifty years of research and applications in reminiscence and life review: State of the art and new directions. *J. Aging Stud.* **2014**, *29*, 29107–29114. [CrossRef] [PubMed]
33. AHTA Definitions and Positions. Available online: https://ahta.memberclicks.net/assets/docs/final_ht_position_paper_updated_409.pdf (accessed on 1 November 2023).
34. Jaidi, Y.; Nonnonhou, V.; Kanagaratnam, L.; Bertholon, L.A.; Badr, S.; Noel, V.; Novella, J.-L.; Mahmoudi, R. Reduction of the anticholinergic burden makes it possible to decrease behavioral and psychological symptoms of dementia. *Am. J. Geriatr. Psychiatry* **2018**, *26*, 280–288. [CrossRef] [PubMed]
35. Beier, M.T. Pharmacotherapy for behavioral and psychological symptoms of dementia in the elderly. *Am. J. Health-Syst. Pharm.* **2007**, *64*, S9–S17. [CrossRef] [PubMed]
36. Press, D.; Alexander, M. *Management of Neuropsychiatric Symptoms of Dementia*; UpToDate: Waltham, MA, USA, 2014; Volume 3, p. 20.
37. Wilson, E.O. *Biophilia*; Harvard University Press: Cambridge, MA, USA, 1984.

38. Gaekwad, J.S.; Sal Moslehian, A.; Roös, P.B.; Walker, A. A meta-analysis of emotional evidence for the biophilia hypothesis and implications for biophilic design. *Front. Psychol.* **2022**, *13*, 750245. [CrossRef]
39. Kaplan, S. The restorative effects of nature: Toward an integrative framework. *J. Environ. Psychol.* **1995**, *15*, 169–182. [CrossRef]
40. Haller, R.L.; Kramer, C.L. *Horticultural Therapy Methods: Making Connections in Health Care, Human Service, and Community Programs*; Haworth: New York, NY, USA, 2006.
41. Smith, B.C.; D'Amico, M. Sensory-Based Interventions for Adults with Dementia and Alzheimer's Disease: A Scoping Review. *Occup. Ther. Health Care* **2020**, *34*, 171–201. [CrossRef] [PubMed]
42. Taylor, A.F.; Kuo, F.; Sullivan, W.C. Coping with ADD: The surprising connection to green play settings. *Environ. Behav.* **2001**, *33*, 54–77. [CrossRef]
43. Wichrowski, M.; Whiteson, J.; Haas, F.; Mola, A.; Rey, M.J. Effects of horticultural therapy on mood and heart rate in patients participating in an inpatient cardiopulmonary rehabilitation program. *J. Cardiopulm. Rehabil.* **2005**, *25*, 270–274. [CrossRef]
44. Waliczek, T.M.; Zajicek, J.M.; Lineberger, R.D. The influence of gardening activities on perceptions of life satisfaction. *Hortic. Sci.* **2005**, *40*, 1360–1365. [CrossRef]
45. Cooper Marcus, C.; Barnes, M. *Healing Gardens*; John Wiley & Sons: New York, NY, USA, 1999.
46. Smith, D.; Aldous, D.E. Effect of therapeutic horticulture on the self-concept of the mildly intellectually disabled student. In *The Healing Dimensions of People-Plant Relations*; Francis, M., Lindsey, P., Stone Rice, J., Eds.; People-Plant Council: San Francisco, CA, USA, 1994; p. 12.
47. Pothukuchi, K.; Bikes, J. *Youth Nutrition Gardens in Detroit: A Report on Benefits, Potential, and Challenges*; Wayne State University: Detroit, MI, USA, 2001.
48. Matsuo, E. Horticulture helps us to live as human beings: Providing balance and harmony in our behavior and thought and life worth living. *Acta Hortic.* **1995**, *391*, 19–30. [CrossRef]
49. Jo, H.; Song, C.; Miyazaki, Y. Physiological benefits of viewing nature: A systematic review of indoor experiments. *Int. J. Environ. Res. Public Health* **2019**, *16*, 4739. [CrossRef]
50. Gardens That Care: Planning Outdoor Environments for People with Dementia. Available online: https://www.enablingenvironments.com.au/uploads/5/0/4/5/50459523/gardens_that_care.planning_outdoor_environments_for_people_with_dementia.pdf (accessed on 30 October 2023).
51. Chalfont, G. *Design for Nature in Dementia Care*; Jessica Kingsley: West Yorkshire, UK, 2007.
52. Sachs, N.; Marcus, C. *Therapeutic Landscapes: An Evidence-Based Approach to Designing Healing Gardens and Restorative Outdoor Spaces*; John Wiley and Sons: Hoboken, NJ, USA, 2014.
53. van der Velde-van Buuringen, M.; Hendriks-van der Sar, R.; Verbeek, H.; Achterberg, W.P.; Caljouw, M.A. The effect of garden use on quality of life and behavioral and psychological symptoms of dementia in people living with dementia in nursing homes: A systematic review. *Front. Psychiatr.* **2023**, *14*, 1044271. [CrossRef]
54. Greenleaf, A.T. Gardens and well-being. In *Encyclopedia of Quality of Life and Well-Being Research*; Michalos, A.C., Ed.; Springer: Dordrecht, The Netherlands, 2014; Volume 1, pp. 2391–2405. [CrossRef]
55. Eldergrow Garden Planting Manual Addendum. 2022. Available online: https://www.dropbox.com/s/ukphr7hqo7rzfqk/Eldergrow%20Educator%20Handbook%20Addendum%20-%20Kickoff%20(KO)%20071222.pdf?dl=0 (accessed on 29 January 2024).
56. D'Andrea, F.; Tischler, V.; Dening, T.; Churchill, A. Olfactory stimulation for people with dementia: A rapid review. *Dementia* **2022**, *5*, 1800–1824. [CrossRef]
57. Her, J.; Cho, M.-K. Effect of aromatherapy on sleep quality of adults and elderly people: A systematic literature review and meta-analysis. *Complement. Ther. Med.* **2021**, *60*, 102739. [CrossRef] [PubMed]
58. Mantle, D.; Pickering, A.T.; Perry, A.K. Medicinal plant extracts for the treatment of dementia: A review of their pharmacology, efficacy and tolerability. *CNS Drugs* **2000**, *13*, 201–213. [CrossRef]
59. Moscovici, M. Horticultural Therapy Activities for Transplant Patients. *J. Ther. Hortic.* **2023**, *33*, 61–79.

Disclaimer/Publisher's Note: The statements, opinions and data contained in all publications are solely those of the individual author(s) and contributor(s) and not of MDPI and/or the editor(s). MDPI and/or the editor(s) disclaim responsibility for any injury to people or property resulting from any ideas, methods, instructions or products referred to in the content.

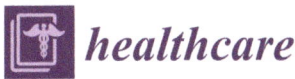

Article

A Brief mHealth-Based Psychological Intervention in Emotion Regulation to Promote Positive Subjective Well-Being in Cardiovascular Disease Patients: A Non-Randomized Controlled Trial

Naima Z. Farhane-Medina [1,2], Rosario Castillo-Mayén [1,2], Bárbara Luque [1,2,*], Sebastián J. Rubio [1,3], Tamara Gutiérrez-Domingo [1,2], Esther Cuadrado [1,2], Alicia Arenas [1,4] and Carmen Tabernero [1,5]

1. Maimonides Biomedical Research Institute of Cordoba (IMIBIC), 14071 Córdoba, Spain
2. Department of Psychology, University of Cordoba, 14071 Córdoba, Spain
3. Department of Didactics of Experimental Sciences, University of Cordoba, 14071 Córdoba, Spain
4. Department of Psychology, University of Seville, 41018 Seville, Spain
5. Institute of Neurosciences of Castilla y León (INCYL), University of Salamanca, 37007 Salamanca, Spain
* Correspondence: bluque@uco.es; Tel.: +34-957-21-89-61

Abstract: The emotional impact that a cardiovascular disease may have on a person's life can affect the prognosis and comorbidity of the disease. Therefore, emotion regulation is most important for the management of the disease. The aim of this study was to analyze the effectiveness of a brief mHealth psychological intervention in emotion regulation to promote positive subjective well-being in cardiovascular disease patients. The study sample ($N = 69$, 63.7 ± 11.5 years) was allocated to either the experimental group ($n = 34$) or control group ($n = 35$). The intervention consisted of a psychoeducational session in emotion regulation and an mHealth-based intervention for 2 weeks. Positive subjective well-being as a primary outcome and self-efficacy to manage the disease as a secondary outcome were assessed at five time points evaluated over a period of 6 weeks. The experimental group showed higher improvement in positive subjective well-being and self-efficacy for managing the disease compared to the control group over time. The experimental group also improved after the intervention on all outcome measures. Brief mHealth interventions in emotion regulation might be effective for improving positive subjective well-being and self-efficacy to manage the disease in cardiovascular patients.

Keywords: cardiovascular disease; positive subjective well-being; emotion regulation; brief psychological intervention; mHealth

1. Introduction

The prevalence of cardiovascular disease (CVD) seems to be stable over time, being the first cause of death and a major loss of health worldwide [1,2]. Empiric evidence has proven that the risk of developing CVD comes not only from biological factors but also from behavioral, psychological, and social factors, which, according to a biopsychosocial model of health, interact with each other [3]. In the same way, the consequences or repercussions of CVD involve the daily life of the people who suffer it, their quality of life, and the emotional balance to cope with it [4]. Therefore, depression [5], anxiety, and stress [6] may appear after CVD. This could be a result of coping with the chronic disease in itself, as well as a consequence of the multi-level changes that these patients have to face after the diagnosis. Comorbid anxiety-depressive symptomatology may complicate their recovery [7] and can also affect their self-efficacy for managing the disease, resulting in the abandonment of medical recommendations, putting their health at risk. Consequently, psychological interventions are needed in order to help patients regulate these emotions in a healthy manner to prevent comorbidity and promote a healthy quality of life. Thus, the purpose

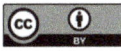

of this study is to develop and test a brief mHealth-based psychological intervention in emotion regulation to promote positive subjective well-being and self-efficacy for managing the disease in CVD patients.

1.1. Brief Psychological Interventions

There are already studies that have incorporated brief psychological interventions into cardiac rehabilitation [8,9]. Their low cost and promising results that seem to have lasting benefits [10–12] place this type of intervention as an interesting supplement to be considered when treating patients with CVD [13]. The chronic nature of this disease implies the need to adopt healthy habits on a continuous basis. The difficulty of modifying lifestyle and adherence to treatment is added to the anxiety-depressive symptomatology as possible conditioning factors for the physical vulnerability of a cardiac pathology [14,15]. Brief psychological interventions improve the prognosis of cardiac rehabilitation, helping patients to adapt to the long-term challenges related to CVD [8]. This kind of intervention appears to have a positive effect in this sense, enhancing psychological well-being, reducing anxiety and depressive symptoms, encouraging the promotion of healthy habits, promoting awareness of the disease, and controlling risk factors [8,9].

1.2. Emotion Regulation and Positive Well-Being

Healthy emotion regulation is crucial for psychological functioning and may be one variable that can also help to protect health and, indirectly, to promote self-efficacy [16]. Historically, emotional psychological interventions have been focused on regulating negative and unpleasant emotions such as depressive and anxious symptoms. However, health and positive psychology have promoted an alternative approach that places positive emotions as the axis of change in these interventions [17]. Related to that, some studies have pointed to an association between positive well-being (i.e., positive affect) and a lower risk of a CVD event [18,19]. In particular, positive well-being has been found to be associated with lower odds of stroke [20], myocardial infarction, and the reduced probability of the recurrence of CVD [21,22]. Positive affect is also related to other CVD characteristics, such as biological responses that may be health protective, lower blood pressure, a lower level of cortisol, and less physiological activation [23–25]. Other studies indicate that the physiological reactivity to positive emotions acts as a counterbalance to the harmful reactivity of negative emotions, for example, helping patients to overcome the psychological consequences, including unpleasant emotions, after a CVD event [26,27]. From this positive perspective, a relationship is established between emotional well-being, focusing on positive emotions, and improving the emotional state of patients with CVD with better development and management of CVD [28].

Given the importance of experiencing positive emotions, having greater positive well-being, and the common anxiety-depression comorbidity [29], emotion regulation intervention oriented to CVD patients becomes highly recommended. Gross defined emotion regulation as "the processes by which individuals influence the emotions they have, when they have them and how they experience and express these emotions" [29], which includes the process of the identification, recognition, acceptance, and normalization of emotions. Healthy emotion regulation becomes critical to coping with challenging situations [30] such as a cardiac event. Even though there is not a lot of research that analyzes the relationship between emotion regulation and CVD, its influence on how patients with CVD deal with their disease seems clear. On the one hand, research has shown that patients with CVD had lower emotion regulation, which can, in some way, be negative to the prognosis of this chronic disease [16,31]. The use of unhealthy emotion regulation strategies may be responsible for the appearance of cardiovascular risk factors, such as body mass index, unhealthy diet, heavy alcohol consumption, sedentariness, etc. [16,32]. On the other hand, people diagnosed with CVD could be prone to deficits in emotion regulation [31]; hence, they would become more vulnerable to developing a mood disorder [33]. Then, for this bidirectional risk between emotional dysregulation and

CVD risk factors, a psychological intervention to promote healthy emotional regulation seems necessary to decrease the odds of developing comorbid problems and, consequently, improve the quality of life of CVD patients.

1.3. mHealth

The term mHealth (mobile health) refers to the use of mobile devices, tablets, health-related applications, and other wireless technologies in health services, medical care, and clinical practice [34]. The incorporation of mHealth strategies aims to facilitate prescribing, adherence, patient communication, and health outcomes [34,35]. Currently, it has stimulated the use of mHealth tools, especially for risk groups such as CVD patients that may have some difficulties attending regular hospital follow-ups [36]. The unstoppable growth of the use of new technologies by the adult population favors the insertion of new techniques to promote, prevent, and intervene in health. The low adherence to treatment for CVD [37], which is probably due to its chronic nature, raises the need for interventions within the reach of these patients [38]. The evidence for this type of intervention is ambiguous so far. On the one hand, there is research that shows poor evidence of the effect of mHealth interventions to improve adherence to treatment (management and medication) in patients with CVD [39,40]. On the other hand, there are studies that point out the potential of mHealth to improve the adherence and management of chronic diseases [41] such as CVD [42]. This kind of intervention has also shown improvements in the physical and mental well-being of patients [43], favoring the management of depressive and anxiety symptoms [44].

1.4. The Present Study

The evidence reviewed above supports the relevance of incorporating an emotional psychological perspective to intervene with CVD patients. It also highlights the cost-effectiveness of brief psychological interventions, together with the promising results of the incorporation of mHealth strategies into healthcare. However, the literature addressing CVD interventions combining these components remains scarce. Therefore, the main aim of this study was to evaluate the effectiveness of a brief mHealth-based psychological intervention in emotion regulation to improve positive subjective well-being (enhancing positive affect) as well as self-efficacy for managing the disease in patients diagnosed with CVD. The first hypothesis was that participants included in the experimental group would have significantly greater positive subjective well-being and better self-efficacy for managing their chronic/cardiac disease compared to the control group. A secondary objective was to test if the expected differences between the groups would be maintained over time. Therefore, the second hypothesis was that better outcomes in positive subjective well-being and in self-efficacy for managing their chronic/cardiac disease in the experimental group would also appear in the follow-up evaluations.

2. Methods

2.1. Study Design

This was an interventional study, specifically, a two-arm non-randomized controlled prospective trial. The experimental group received a psychoeducational session in emotion regulation and a subsequent brief mHealth-based psychological intervention in emotion regulation, while the control group continued with their treatment as usual. The study was approved by the Andalusian Health Service's Research Ethics Committee and the Reina Sofía Hospital in June 2015 (Acta 242, Ref. 2886, 29 June 2015).

2.2. Participants

Participants diagnosed with any type of CVD (angina pectoris, myocardial infarction, heart failure, arrhythmia, etc.) were recruited between March 2019 and April 2019 from the Cardiology Unit of Reina Sofía University Hospital of Córdoba, Spain. The inclusion criteria were: (1) women and men with a diagnosis of a CVD aged > 18, (2) ability to be fluent in Spanish, (3) having a smartphone compatible with the app used for the mHealth intervention (*WhatsApp*) and daily access to the internet, (4) having the required digital skills to follow the mHealth intervention, (5) not currently participating in another clinical trial, and (6) not currently receiving other psychological treatment. The exclusion criteria were: (1) women and men with a diagnosis of a CVD < 18 years, (2) not fluent in Spanish, (3) not having a smartphone compatible with the app used for the mHealth intervention and daily access to the internet, (4) not having the required digital skills, (5) serious mental health condition, (6) currently participating in another clinical trial, and (7) currently receiving other psychological treatment.

Potential participants ($N = 132$) were approached by telephone by an assistant researcher. Sixty-nine patients ($M = 63.70$ years, $SD = 11.50$) met the inclusion criteria and agreed to participate in the study, giving their informed consent. The participants were assigned to either the experimental group ($n = 34$) or the control group ($n = 35$) depending on their availability to attend the face-to-face session. There were seven dropouts and one death. Finally, 61 patients remained and completed all the study phases. The sociodemographic characteristics of the sample are described in Table 1.

2.3. Procedure

2.3.1. Experimental Group

The experimental condition included a one-and-only face-to-face emotion regulation psychoeducational session and a subsequent mHealth-based emotion regulation psychological intervention.

Psychoeducational session. It was performed by a General Health psychologist in a private room at the Clinical Research Building of the Maimonides Biomedical Research Institute of Cordoba in small groups of about two to four people and lasted 60 min. The aim of this face-to-face session was psychoeducation about emotions, including identification, recognition, acceptance, and regulation, in order to facilitate the following mHealth intervention. Therefore, the session was structured in accordance with the above-mentioned objectives following the next headings and content: (a) What are emotions? Description and explanation of emotions concept, (b) Differences between basic and complex emotions: Provision of information about the different types of emotions regarding its nature, (c) Function and structure of emotions: Analyzing the function of emotions on a daily basis and, (d) Emotion regulation: Psychoeducation about the emotion regulation strategies, more specifically related to the management of their CVD diagnosis and provision of resources to improve emotion regulation.

In this session, two evaluations were conducted: the pre-test evaluation (baseline measurements) and after the psychoeducational session (post-session). In order to promote the intervention adherence, the patients were given a description of the mHealth intervention procedure with some motivational messages reinforcing their participation at the end of the session.

mHealth intervention. It started the day after the face-to-face session. The patients received for the next 14 days a *WhatsApp* message every day at the same time with an emotion regulation activity they had to perform (Supplementary File S1). The program of activities was based on Leahy et al. [45]. The order and content of the messages followed the scheme explained in the face-to-face session: the identification, recognition, acceptance, and regulation of emotions. The messages were prepared to be as brief and understandable as possible to be in accordance with brief psychological interventions.

After this intervention, the effectiveness of the mHealth intervention was evaluated (post-mHealth). To assess the changes, if any were maintained over time, two follow-up evaluations were included 2 weeks (follow-up 1) and 4 weeks (follow-up 2) after the mHealth intervention.

2.3.2. Control Group

The participants of this group continued their regular medical follow-up without attending the psychoeducational session or receiving the mHealth intervention.

Thus, each participant of the experimental group was assessed at five different time points (baseline, post-session, post-mHealth, follow-up 1, and follow-up 2), whilst the participants of the control group were evaluated four times (baseline, post-mHealth, follow-up 1, and follow-up 2, Figure 1). The baseline and post-session evaluations of the experimental group were measured in situ through an online questionnaire. The baseline measurements of the control group, as well as the three post-evaluations (post-mHealth, follow-up 1, and follow-up 2) of both groups were conducted by phone calls.

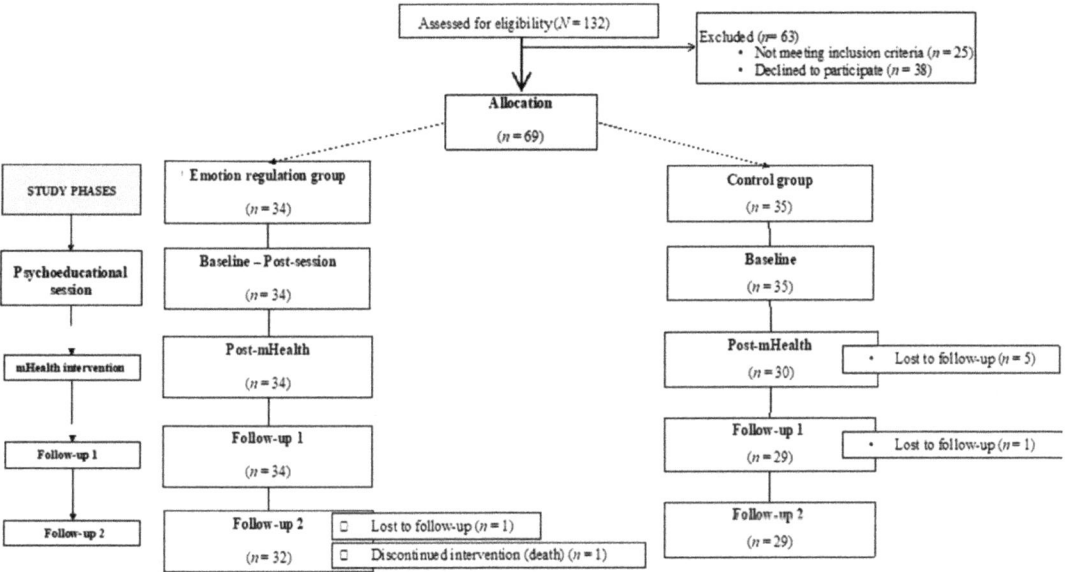

Figure 1. Flow chart of the sample and phases of the study.

2.4. Outcome Measures

2.4.1. Participant Characteristics

Sociodemographic characteristics including, age, sex, marital status, employment status, educational level, as well as the type of CVD and the level of limitation on activities of daily living (ADL) were asked of the participants. In addition, relevant psychological variables to the aim of the intervention, anxiety, and depression states and positivity, were also assessed to complete the description of the study sample. The scales used were the Spanish-validated version of the Hospital Anxiety and Depression Scale—HADS [46,47] (e.g., anxiety: Worrying thoughts go through my mind; depression: I still enjoy the things I used to enjoy)—and the Spanish-validated version of the Positivity Scale—P-scale [48] (e.g., I have great faith in the future).

2.4.2. Primary Outcome
Positive Subjective Well-Being (PSWB)

It was assessed through the Positive Affect subscale (PA), from PANAS [49], the brief Spanish version [50]. The PA is a 10-item Likert-type scale that assesses to what extent participants experience pleasant emotions (e.g., To what extent do you feel interest [enthusiasm, inspiration]). The items are rated from 1 (not at all) to 5 (very much). The value for Cronbach's alpha in the original study was 0.88 for this subscale. In this sample, the reliability value was α = 0.88 too.

2.4.3. Secondary Outcome

Self-Efficacy for Managing the Disease. To provide a more complete evaluation of this outcome, it was assessed by means of two instruments that measure different types of disease management self-efficacy:

Self-Efficacy for Managing Chronic Disease (SEMCD—Spanish validated version) [51]. This Likert-type scale assesses self-efficacy for managing a chronic disease. It is composed of six items (e.g., How confident do you feel that you can keep the emotional distress caused by your disease from interfering with the things you want to do?) rated from 1 = (not at all confident) to 10 (totally confident). In the original study, Cronbach's alpha coefficient was 0.85, and in this study sample, it was α = 0.86.

Cardiovascular Management Self-Efficacy Scale (CMSES—Spanish translated version) [52]. The CMSES was used to evaluate the perceived self-efficacy to manage the CVD. The CMSES is composed of nine items divided into three factors: cardiac risk (e.g., How well can you avoid problems or difficult situations and reduce sources of stress?), adherence to treatment (e.g., How well can you follow the prescriptions about food, even when you feel very nervous), and the recognition of cardiac symptomatology (e.g., How well can you recognize illness symptoms, such as palpitations, tachycardia, and short breath?). It uses a Likert-type scale of 5 points, from 1 (not at all confident) to 5 (totally confident). The reliability in the original study was α = 0.68; in this sample, it was 0.71.

In addition to the instruments mentioned above, a specific scale was created to obtain a subjective evaluation of the intervention at each phase of the study from the participants of the experimental group. This was a Likert-type scale composed of three items regarding adherence to the intervention, satisfaction with the intervention, and a general evaluation. The adherence to the intervention was measured in terms of frequency in reading and following the instructions of the mHealth intervention, from 1 (never) to 5 (every day). The degree of satisfaction with the messages received was evaluated from 1 (not at all satisfied) to 5 (completely satisfied), and finally, the general evaluation of the study was assessed from 1 (not at all satisfied) to 5 (completely satisfied). Cronbach's alpha value for this scale was 0.75.

2.5. Data Analysis

The sample size was calculated using the G*Power 3.1.9.6 program [53] based on a previous study [54]. This study required a minimum of 34 participants in total to maintain a significance level of 0.05, an effect size of 0.25, and a power of 80.0%. The whole sample comprised 69 participants considering a dropout rate higher than 20% [55].

Student's *t*-test, the chi-square test, and Fisher's exact test were performed to compare the sociodemographic and clinical characteristics between groups. A dependent sample *t*-test was conducted to test if there were differences before and after the psychoeducational session for the experimental group. To test the effect of the intervention, a repeated-measures ANOVA was performed with each study variable with Time as a within-subject factor (baseline, post-mHealth, follow-up 1, and follow-up 2) and the experimental condition as a between-subject factor (experimental vs. control group). Bonferroni correction was used for pairwise comparisons. The data were analyzed using SPSS statistic software (v. 28).

3. Results

Table 1 shows the sociodemographic and clinical characteristics of the study sample. Statistically significant differences between groups were only found for employment status ($p = 0.004$). The baseline scores for each group on all outcome measures are shown in Table 2. No differences were found between the groups.

Table 1. Participant sociodemographic and clinical characteristics of the study sample.

	Total (N = 69)	Experimental Group (n = 34)	Control Group (n = 35)	Statistical Significance
Age (M, SD)	63.7 (11.5)	61.24 (11.1)	66.1 (11.6)	$t(67) = 1.77, p = 0.081$ [a]
Sex, n (%)				$\chi^2(1) = 1.95, p = 0.163$ [b]
Male	54 (78.3%)	29	25	
Female	15 (21.7%)	5	10	
Marital status, n (%)				$p = 0.924$ [c]
Single	2 (2.9%)	1	1	
Single with partner	1 (1.4%)	1	0	
Married	57 (82.6%)	28	29	
Separated	2 (2.9%)	1	1	
Divorced	3 (4.3%)	2	1	
Widowed	4 (5.8%)	1	3	
Employment status, n (%)				$p = 0.004$ [c]
Retired	40 (58%)	13	27	
Full-time work	21 (30.4%)	15	6	
Unemployed	6 (8.7%)	5	1	
Home care	2 (2.9%)	1	1	
Educational level, n (%)				$p = 0.119$ [c]
Basic primary school	54 (78.3%)	24	30	
High school or higher	15 (21.7%)	10	5	
Type of CVD, n (%)				$p = 0.677$ [c]
Angina pectoris	8 (11.6%)	3	5	
Myocardial infarction	33 (47.8%)	17	16	
Heart failure	5 (7.3%)	1	4	
Arrhythmia	5 (7.3%)	2	3	
Other	11 (15.9%)	7	4	
More than one of the above	7 (10.1)	4	3	
Level of limitation of ADLs, n (%)				
Level 1	29 (42%)	17	12	
Level 2	22 (31.9%)	10	12	
Level 3	14 (20.3%)	4	10	
Level 4	4 (5.8%)	3	1	
HADS (M, SD)	1.84 (0.49)	1.95 (0.44)	1.73 (0.52)	$t(65) = -1.88, p = 0.065$ [a]
P-scale (M, SD)	3.94 (0.82)	3.89 (0.69)	3.99 (0.93)	$t(67) = 0.50, p = 0.614$ [a]

Note. M = mean, SD = standard deviation, ADLs = activities of daily living, CVD = cardiovascular disease, HADS = Hospital Anxiety and Depression Scale, P-scale = Positivity scale. [a] Student's t-test, [b] Chi-square test, [c] Fisher's exact Test.

Table 2. Baseline scores in the experimental and the control group in all the outcome measures.

	Experimental Group (n = 34)		Control Group (n = 35)		
	M	SD	M	SD	p
PSWB	3.28	0.76	3.36	0.85	0.674
SEMCD	7.71	1.79	6.85	1.92	0.059
CMSES	4.11	0.66	4.31	0.47	0.144

Note. M = mean, SD = standard deviation, PSWB = Positive Subjective Well-Being, SEMCD = Self-Efficacy for Managing Chronic Disease, CMSES = Cardiovascular Management Self-Efficacy Scale.

3.1. Psychoeducational Session

Table 3 shows the means, standard deviations, and *t*-test results of PSWB, SEMCD, and CMSES at the baseline and after the face-to-face session for the intervention group. The results from dependent *t*-test analysis showed differences between these two phases in positive subjective well-being and self-efficacy for managing the CVD, with higher scores in both scales in the post-session evaluation compared to the baseline.

Table 3. Baseline and post-session scores of PSWB, SEMCD, and CMSES in the experimental group.

	Baseline		Post-Session (Face-to-Face)		Baseline–Post-Session Emotion Regulation		
	M	SD	M	SD	t(33)	p	d
PSWB	3.28	0.76	3.93	0.68	−6.60	<0.001	0.57
SEMCD	7.71	1.79	8.02	2.00	−1.40	0.170	1.31
CMSES	4.11	0.66	4.26	0.67	−2.42	0.021	0.35

Note. *M* = mean, *SD* = standard deviation, PSWB = Positive Subjective Well-Being, SEMCD = Self-Efficacy for Managing Chronic Disease, CMSES = Cardiovascular Management Self-Efficacy Scale.

3.2. mHealth Intervention

The graphics presented in Figures 2–4 show the marginal estimated means for both groups at the baseline and at the three post-test measures on PSWB, CMSES, and SEMCD.

3.2.1. Primary Outcome

Positive Subjective Well-being (PSWB)

The repeated-measures ANOVA showed a significant main effect of time [$F(3177) = 13.60$, $p < 0.001$, $\eta p^2 = 0.19$, observed power (OP) = 1.00], and a significant interaction effect of time x experimental condition [$F(3177) = 4.70$, $p = 0.003$, $\eta p^2 = 0.07$, OP = 0.89]. Bonferroni pairwise comparisons showed significant differences between groups at post-mHealth ($M_{experimental} = 4.01$, $M_{control} = 3.48$, $p = 0.008$; 95% IC = [0.14, −0.92]), and follow-up 2 ($M_{experimental} = 4.01$, $M_{control} = 3.59$, $p = 0.035$; 95% IC = [0.03, 0.81]). Additionally, within the experimental group, some differences were found in PSWB between the study phases, being the scores higher in all post-evaluations compared to the baseline (all $ps < 0.001$).

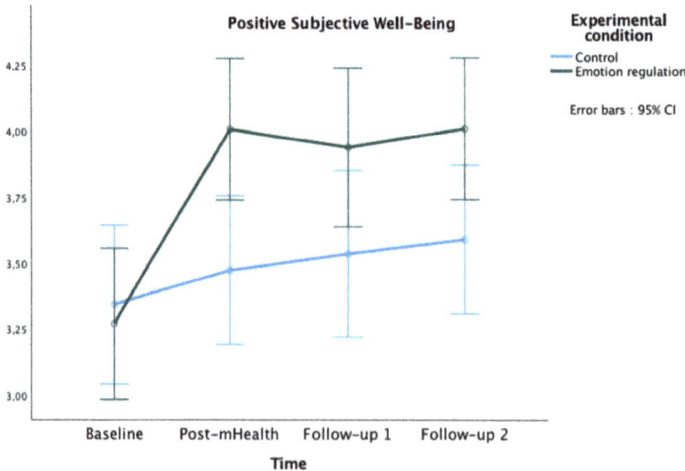

Figure 2. Changes in Positive Subjective Well-being in both groups over time.

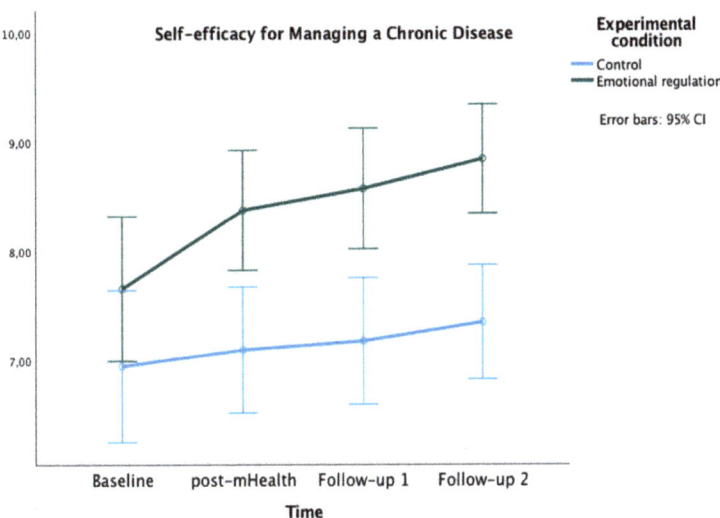

Figure 3. Changes in Self-efficacy for Managing Chronic Disease in both groups over time.

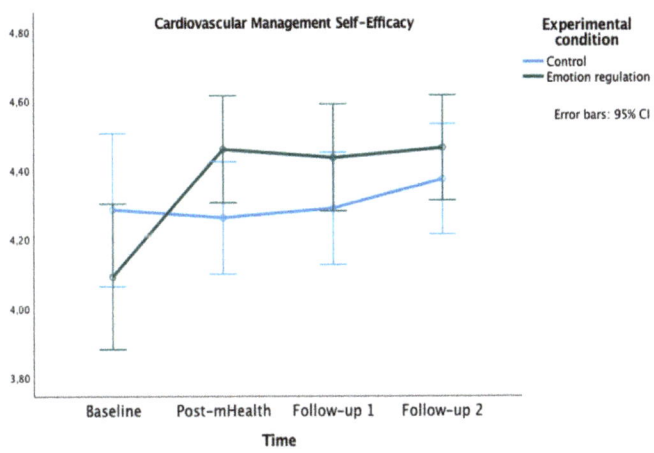

Figure 4. Changes in Cardiac Management Self-Efficacy in both groups over time.

3.2.2. Secondary Outcome

Self-Efficacy for Managing the Disease

With regard to the SEMCD, a significant main effect of time was found [$F(2.585, 152.50) = 7.27$, $p < 0.01$, $\eta p^2 = 0.11$, potency = 0.97, Greenhouse-Geisser correction applied because Mauchly's $W = 0.759$, $p = 0.007$]. Additionally, a main effect of the experimental condition was found [$F(1) = 12.04$, $p = 0.001$, $\eta p^2 = 0.17$, OP = 0.93]. Bonferroni pairwise comparisons showed significant differences between groups at post-mHealth ($M_{experimental} = 8.38$, $M_{control} = 7.10$, $p = 0.002$; 95% IC = [0.48, 2.07]), follow-up 1 ($M_{experimental} = 8.57$, $M_{control} = 7.19$, $p = 0.001$; 95% IC = [0.60, 2.20]), and follow-up 2 ($M_{experimental} = 8.84$, $M_{control} = 7.35$, $p < 0.001$; 95% IC = [0.77, 2.22]). Within the experimental group, differences were also found with higher scores on SEMCD at all post-evaluations compared to the baseline (all $ps < 0.05$).

Related to the CMSES, a significant main effect of time [$F(2.45, 144.74) = 6.40$, $p < 0.001$, $\eta p^2 = 0.10$, OP = 0.94] and an interaction effect of time x experimental condition [$F(2.45$,

144.74) = 4.91, p = 0.005, ηp^2 = 0.08, OP = 0.86] were found. In both cases, the Greenhouse–Geisser correction was applied because Mauchly's W = 0.70, p = 0.001. Bonferroni pairwise comparisons were not significant. However, the experimental group showed higher values on CMSES at post-mHealth (M = 4.46), follow-up 1 (M = 4.43) and follow-up 2 (M = 4.46) compared to the baseline (M = 4.09), all ps = 0.001.

3.3. Subjective Evaluation of the Intervention

The results indicated a great commitment and a positive evaluation of the intervention, showing differences over the three time point evaluations [$F(2,62)$ = 15.5, p < 0.001, ηp^2 = 0.33, OP = 0.99]. Specifically, the results showed improvements in each phase, comparing post-mHealth (M = 4.27), follow-up 1 (M = 4.44), and follow-up 2 (M = 4.69), all ps < 0.05.

4. Discussion

The aim of this study was to evaluate the effectiveness of an mHealth-based brief psychological intervention in emotion regulation to enhance positive subjective well-being and self-efficacy to manage the chronic cardiac disease in patients with CVD. The study sample of 69 CVD patients (54 men, 15 women) was assigned to either the experimental (n = 34) or the control group (n = 35). Both groups were composed mostly of men in line with the sex distribution in CVD patients [56]. A face-to-face psychoeducational session followed by an mHealth intervention was conducted. Regarding the effectiveness of the face-to-face session, the results showed remarkable differences. The 1 h psychological intervention in emotion regulation strongly improved the patients' positive subjective well-being. Moreover, this face-to-face session seemed to increase their perception of self-efficacy in managing the CVD. The mHealth emotion regulation intervention improved the positive subjective well-being of patients, as well as provided better management of the disease compared to the control group. According to the hypotheses of the study, the results showed a higher positive subjective well-being across the evaluations and a better cardiac and chronic management self-efficacy comparing both follow-ups with the baseline. Important differences over time were also found between the groups. The experimental group showed a greater positive subjective well-being in post-mHealth and follow-up 2, and a higher self-efficacy for managing chronic disease in post-mHealth, follow-up 1, and follow-up 2 compared to the control group.

These results corroborate those obtained by other studies, backing up the effectiveness of emotion regulation in improving psychological well-being [57–59]. The present results further suggest the effectiveness of psychological interventions in improving well-being in patients with CVD, according to previous research findings [28], as well as in enhancing self-efficacy in patients with CVD. These results are in line with several studies that analyzed the connection between positive affect, psychological well-being, and the management of CVD. Some of them found that patients with higher subjective well-being were prone to have healthier habits, such as taking care of diet, better sleep quality, reduced alcohol consumption, and better adherence to treatment [22,60–62], resulting in lower CVD risk [20,22].

Results from this study are consistent with research findings that highlight the importance of implementing emotion regulation techniques with patients who manifest cardiovascular problems [16,57,63] in order to favor healthy physical and psychological functioning, as well as reduce cardiovascular risk. Moreover, according to this study, an mHealth-based brief psychological intervention seems to be at least a good start to achieve these benefits in this population. This would not only be because of the increased subjective positive well-being, which would have already led to an improvement in quality of life and other health-related variables [64] but also because it has an effect, at least at the middle term, on the management of cardiac and chronic disease. Therefore, these findings contribute to the growing evidence that regards psychological well-being as a "bulwark" of health [19,20,59]. The significance and maintenance of the intervention effect in both self-efficacy measures and subjective well-being support the existing evidence of the lasting benefits of this brief type of educational intervention [10–12], giving strength to the idea of incorporating this kind of psychological intervention in cardiac rehabilitation programs [8,9].

In addition, as other studies have suggested, the use of new technologies allowed us to reach directly to the *patient's hand*, which may have been one of the reasons for the high adherence to the intervention as shown in the results about the subjective evaluation in the study [41,42]. The effectiveness of a positive brief mHealth psychological intervention could imply a better adaptation to the disease, adherence to treatment, and the adoption of a new healthy lifestyle [8,60,61]. This may suppose an improvement in well-being and quality of life [28], reducing long-term risk factors such as comorbidities [5,6]. The results of this study seem to indicate that the combination of brief psychological interventions, due to their low cost and promptness, together with the adaptation of the treatments to the rising technological reality, are an attractive and effective alternative which can be considered from different approaches of health care when treating these patients [65].

4.1. Limitations

Although the results indicated the effectiveness of the intervention, this study has some limitations. The non-random allocation of the participants on the experimental conditions may bias the results. However, no differences between groups were found in clinical characteristics such as anxiety and depression states, positivity, or any outcome measure at baseline. Regarding the study sample size, though limited, it was similar to previous intervention studies with CVD patients [66,67]. Similar results are expected in wider samples, but this needs to be tested in future research. A potential bias in the data collection also needs to be mentioned. Baseline measurements were conducted differently for the experimental and the control groups (in situ vs. phone call, respectively), which could have affected the study results. However, as mentioned before, no differences between the groups were found at baseline, indicating that the different procedure would have not affected the participants' responses. Finally, the low presence of women in the study sample is consistent with the pattern of a higher prevalence of most CVD in men. However, several studies argue that this sex prevalence ratio is based on a gender bias in the diagnosis of CVD [56]. Relating to that, in our study, the underrepresentation of women is higher in the experimental group (29 men/5 women) compared to the control group (25 men/10 women). This lower enrolment of women in CVD programs has been observed in other studies [68]. This could be explained, among other things, by the underestimation of CVD risk in women, a lower importance of self-care, as well as some gender barriers (e.g., lower social and family support, transport-economic problems, lack of time due to the caregiving role) [69]. Although this issue might bias the results, it is important to note that in our study there were no statistical differences in the sex representation between groups.

4.2. Future Research

Regarding future lines of research, it would be interesting to evaluate and compare the effectiveness of the intervention proposed with other types of intervention modalities (i.e., only face-to-face, only mHealth, and no treatment). This would shed light on the effect of interventions mediated by the incorporation of mHealth strategies. It is also proposed to go one step further and take advantage of the fact that mHealth interventions are projected as a patient-centered strategy to encourage a personalized intervention, a tailored communication, considering the individualities of the patients with regard to the objective of the intervention. In this line, the gender bias mentioned above should be taken into account when designing future interventions in CVD. The personalization of these interventions would allow to address the specific characteristics of women, facilitating their enrolment and hopefully improving their CVD-related outcomes. In addition, other variables could also be evaluated at baseline, considering the gender perspective and the profiles of patients with CVD. Furthermore, the possibility of adding biomarkers in future research should be contemplated in order to obtain richer and likely less-biased information on the intervention.

5. Conclusions

This study shows the effectiveness of an mHealth-based brief psychological intervention in emotion regulation to enhance positive subjective well-being (showing an increase in positive affect) and to improve self-efficacy in the management of chronic and cardiac disease in CVD patients. The adaptation of psychological interventions with new technologies and new forms of understanding life and healthcare treatments was a good option to reach different patient profiles and to promote adherence to the psychological intervention. The results of this study are significant as they provide evidence on how brief psychological interventions together with mHealth are a good combination treatment for CVD patients. It has been proved that with a low cost and promising benefits, together they can contribute to an improvement in psychological well-being and the management of the disease that may translate in the long term to a better quality of life of CVD patients.

Supplementary Materials: The following supporting information can be downloaded at: https://www.mdpi.com/article/10.3390/healthcare10091640/s1, Supplementary File S1: WhatsApp Messages from the mHealth Intervention.

Author Contributions: Conceptualization, R.C.-M., B.L. and C.T.; Data curation, N.Z.F.-M. and T.G.-D.; Formal analysis, N.Z.F.-M., R.C.-M. and B.L.; Funding acquisition, B.L. and C.T.; Investigation, N.Z.F.-M., R.C.-M., B.L., S.J.R., T.G.-D., E.C., A.A. and C.T.; Methodology, R.C.-M., B.L. and C.T.; Project administration, B.L. and C.T.; Resources, B.L. and C.T.; Software, S.J.R.; Supervision, R.C.-M., B.L. and C.T.; Validation, N.Z.F.-M., R.C.-M., B.L., S.J.R., T.G.-D., E.C., A.A. and C.T.; Visualization, N.Z.F.-M., R.C.-M., B.L., S.J.R., T.G.-D., E.C., A.A. and C.T.; Writing—original draft, N.Z.F.-M.; Writing—review and editing, N.Z.F.-M., R.C.-M., B.L. and C.T. All authors have read and agreed to the published version of the manuscript.

Funding: This research was funded by the Spanish Ministry of Economy and Competitiveness, grant number PSI2014-58609-R, and by the Spanish Ministry of Science, Innovation and Universities, grant number PDI2019-107304RB-I00.

Institutional Review Board Statement: The study was conducted according to the guidelines of the Declaration of Helsinki and approved by the Andalusian Health Service's Research Ethics Committee and the Reina Sofía Hospital in June 2015 (Acta 242, ref 2886, 29 June 2015).

Informed Consent Statement: Informed consent was obtained from all subjects involved in the study.

Data Availability Statement: The data presented in this study are available on request from the corresponding author.

Conflicts of Interest: The authors declare no conflict of interest.

References

1. Roth, G.A.; Johnson, C.; Abajobir, A.; Abd-Allah, F.; Abera, S.F.; Abyu, G.; Ahmed, M.; Aksut, B.; Alam, T.; Alam, K.; et al. Global, regional, and national burden of cardiovascular diseases for 10 causes, 1990 to 2015. *J. Am. Coll. Cardiol.* **2017**, *70*, 1–25. [CrossRef]
2. Cardiovascular Diseases. Available online: https://www.who.int/health-topics/cardiovascular-diseases/#tab=tab_1 (accessed on 30 June 2022).
3. Patel, S.; Saha, A.; Poojary, P.; Pandya, D.; Pawar, S.; Patel, J.; Mahajan, K.; Mondal, P.; Agarwal, S.; Hollander, G.; et al. Trends and impact of psychosocial factors in adults with congenital heart disease in the United States. *J. Am. Coll. Cardiol.* **2018**, *71*, A561. [CrossRef]
4. Larkin, K.T.; Chantler, P.D. Chapter 1—Stress, depression, and cardiovascular disease. In *Cardiovascular Implications of Stress and Depression*; Chantler, P.D., Larkin, K.T., Eds.; Academic Press: Cambridge, MA, USA, 2020; pp. 1–12; ISBN 978-0-12-815015-3.
5. Grewal, K.; Gravely-Witte, S.; Stewart, D.E.; Grace, S.L. A simultaneous test of the relationship between identified psychosocial risk factors and recurrent events in coronary artery disease patients. *Anxiety Stress Coping* **2011**, *24*, 463–475. [CrossRef]
6. Grenier, S.; Potvin, O.; Hudon, C.; Boyer, R.; Préville, M.; Desjardins, L.; Bherer, L. Twelve-month prevalence and correlates of subthreshold and threshold anxiety in community-dwelling older adults with cardiovascular diseases. *J. Affect. Disord.* **2012**, *136*, 724–732. [CrossRef]

7. Chen, H.; Wang, X.; Huang, Y.; Li, G.; Liu, Z.; Li, Y.; Geng, H. Prevalence, risk factors and multi-group latent class analysis of lifetime anxiety disorders comorbid depressive symptoms. *J. Affect. Disord.* **2019**, *243*, 360–365. [CrossRef]
8. Fernandes, A.C.; McIntyre, T.; Coelho, R.; Prata, J.; Maciel, M.J. Impact of a brief psychological intervention on lifestyle, risk factors and disease knowledge during phase i of cardiac rehabilitation after acute coronary syndrome. *Rev. Port. Cardiol. Engl. Ed.* **2019**, *38*, 361–368. [CrossRef]
9. Fernandes, A.C.; McIntyre, T.; Coelho, R.; Prata, J.; Maciel, M.J. Brief psychological intervention in phase I of cardiac rehabilitation after acute coronary syndrome. *Rev. Port. Cardiol.* **2017**, *36*, 641–649. [CrossRef]
10. Armitage, C.J. A brief psychological intervention to protect subjective well-being in a community sample. *Qual. Life Res.* **2016**, *25*, 385–391. [CrossRef]
11. Cohen, G.L.; Sherman, D.K. The psychology of change: Self-affirmation and social psychological intervention. *Annu. Rev. Psychol.* **2014**, *65*, 333–371. [CrossRef]
12. Garcia, J.; Cohen, G.L. A social psychological approach to educational intervention. In *The Behavioral Foundations of Public Policy*; Princeton University Press: Princeton, NJ, USA, 2013; pp. 329–347. ISBN 978-0-691-13756-8.
13. Abreu, A. Breve intervenção psicológica em doentes internados após síndrome coronária aguda: Essencial ou acessória? *Rev. Port. Cardiol.* **2017**, *36*, 651–654. [CrossRef]
14. Mikkelsen, M.E.; Gaieski, D.F.; Goyal, M.; Miltiades, A.N.; Munson, J.C.; Pines, J.M.; Fuchs, B.D.; Shah, C.V.; Bellamy, S.L.; Christie, J.D. Factors associated with nonadherence to early goal-directed therapy in the ED. *Chest* **2010**, *138*, 551–558. [CrossRef]
15. Van Der Laan, D.M.; Elders, P.J.M.; Boons, C.C.L.M.; Nijpels, G.; Hugtenburg, J.G. Factors associated with nonadherence to cardiovascular medications: A cross-sectional study. *J. Cardiovasc. Nurs.* **2019**, *34*, 344–352. [CrossRef]
16. Appleton, A.A.; Loucks, E.B.; Buka, S.L.; Kubzansky, L.D. Divergent associations of antecedent- and response-focused emotion regulation strategies with midlife cardiovascular disease risk. *Ann. Behav. Med.* **2014**, *48*, 246–255. [CrossRef]
17. Bolier, L.; Haverman, M.; Westerhof, G.J.; Riper, H.; Smit, F.; Bohlmeijer, E. Positive psychology interventions: A meta-analysis of randomized controlled studies. *BMC Public Health* **2013**, *13*, 119. [CrossRef]
18. Boehm, J.K.; Chen, Y.; Koga, H.; Mathur, M.B.; Vie, L.L.; Kubzansky, L.D. Is optimism associated with healthier cardiovascular-related behavior? Meta-analyses of 3 health behaviors. *Circ. Res.* **2018**, *122*, 1119–1134. [CrossRef]
19. Boehm, J.K.; Kubzansky, L.D. The heart's content: The association between positive psychological well-being and cardiovascular health. *Psychol. Bull.* **2012**, *138*, 655–691. [CrossRef]
20. Lambiase, M.J.; Kubzansky, L.D.; Thurston, R.C. Positive psychological health and stroke risk: The benefits of emotional vitality. *Health Psychol.* **2015**, *34*, 1043–1046. [CrossRef]
21. Kim, E.S.; Sun, J.K.; Park, N.; Kubzansky, L.D.; Peterson, C. Purpose in life and reduced risk of myocardial infarction among older U.S. adults with coronary heart disease: A two-year follow-up. *J. Behav. Med.* **2013**, *36*, 124–133. [CrossRef]
22. Sin, N.L. The protective role of positive well-being in cardiovascular disease: Review of current evidence, mechanisms, and clinical implications. *Curr. Cardiol. Rep.* 2016 1811 **2016**, *18*, 106. [CrossRef]
23. Brummett, B.H.; Boyle, S.H.; Kuhn, C.M.; Siegler, I.C.; Williams, R.B. Positive affect is associated with cardiovascular reactivity, norepinephrine level, and morning rise in salivary cortisol. *Psychophysiology* **2009**, *46*, 862–869. [CrossRef]
24. Dockray, S.; Steptoe, A. Positive affect and psychobiological processes. *Neurosci. Biobehav. Rev.* **2010**, *35*, 69–75. [CrossRef]
25. Steptoe, A.; Leigh Gibson, E.; Hamer, M.; Wardle, J. Neuroendocrine and cardiovascular correlates of positive affect measured by ecological momentary assessment and by questionnaire. *Psychoneuroendocrinology* **2007**, *32*, 56–64. [CrossRef]
26. Huffman, J.C.; Beale, E.E.; Celano, C.M.; Beach, S.R.; Belcher, A.M.; Moore, S.V.; Suarez, L.; Motiwala, S.R.; Gandhi, P.U.; Gaggin, H.K.; et al. Effects of optimism and gratitude on physical activity, biomarkers, and readmissions after an acute coronary syndrome: The gratitude research in acute coronary events study. *Circ. Cardiovasc. Qual. Outcomes* **2016**, *9*, 55–63. [CrossRef]
27. Mavaddat, N.; Ross, S.; Dobbin, A.; Williams, K.; Graffy, J.; Mant, J. Training in positivity for stroke? A qualitative study of acceptability of use of positive mental training (PosMT) as a tool to assist stroke survivors with post-stroke psychological problems and in coping with rehabilitation. *NeuroRehabilitation* **2017**, *40*, 259–270. [CrossRef]
28. Sanjuán, P.; Montalbetti, T.; Pérez-García, A.M.; Bermúdez, J.; Arranz, H.; Castro, A. A randomised trial of a positive intervention to promote well-being in cardiac patients. *Appl. Psychol. Health Well-Being* **2016**, *8*, 64–84. [CrossRef]
29. Gross, J.J. The emerging field of emotion regulation: An integrative review. *Rev. Gen. Psychol.* **1998**, *2*, 271–299. [CrossRef]
30. Gross, J.J. Emotion regulation: Taking stock and moving forward. *Emotion* **2013**, *13*, 359–365. [CrossRef]
31. Spitznagel, M.B.; Potter, V.; Miller, L.A.; Roberts Miller, A.N.; Hughes, J.; Rosneck, J.; Gunstad, J. Ability to regulate emotion is predicted by depressive symptoms and cognitive function in a cardiac sample. *J. Cardiovasc. Nurs.* **2013**, *28*, 453–459. [CrossRef]
32. Haedtke, C.; Smith, M.; Vanburen, J.; Klein, D.; Turvey, C. The relationships among pain, depression, and physical activity in patients with heart failure. *J. Cardiovasc. Nurs.* **2017**, *32*, E21–E25. [CrossRef]
33. Bichara, V.M.; Santillán, J.; de Rosa, R.; Estofan, L. Depresión en insuficiencia cardíaca crónica: Causa o consecuencia. *Insuf Card* **2016**, *11*, 173–200.
34. Cruz-Ramos, N.A.; Alor-Hernández, G.; Colombo-Mendoza, L.O.; Sánchez-Cervantes, J.L.; Rodríguez-Mazahua, L.; Guarneros-Nolasco, L.R. MHealth apps for self-management of cardiovascular diseases: A scoping review. *Healthcare* **2022**, *10*, 322. [CrossRef]
35. Malvey, D.; Slovensky, D.J. *MHealth: Transforming Healthcare*; Springer: Berlin/Heidelberg, Germany, 2014, ISBN 978-1-4899-7457-0.

36. Scherrenberg, M.; Wilhelm, M.; Hansen, D.; Völler, H.; Cornelissen, V.; Frederix, I.; Kemps, H.; Dendale, P. The future is now: A call for action for cardiac telerehabilitation in the COVID-19 pandemic from the secondary prevention and rehabilitation section of the european association of preventive cardiology. *Eur. J. Prev. Cardiol.* **2021**, *28*, 524–540. [CrossRef]
37. Chowdhury, R.; Khan, H.; Heydon, E.; Shroufi, A.; Fahimi, S.; Moore, C.; Stricker, B.; Mendis, S.; Hofman, A.; Mant, J.; et al. Adherence to cardiovascular therapy: A meta-analysis of prevalence and clinical consequences. *Eur. Heart J.* **2013**, *34*, 2940–2948. [CrossRef]
38. Klimis, H.; Thakkar, J.; Chow, C.K. Breaking barriers: Mobile health interventions for cardiovascular disease. *Can. J. Cardiol.* **2018**, *34*, 905–913. [CrossRef]
39. Adler, A.J.; Martin, N.; Mariani, J.; Tajer, C.D.; Serrano, N.C.; Casas, J.P.; Perel, P. Mobile phone text messaging to improve adherence to cardiovascular disease secondary prevention interventions. *Cochrane Database Syst. Rev.* **2015**, *2015*. [CrossRef]
40. Palmer, M.J.; Barnard, S.; Perel, P.; Free, C. Mobile phone-based interventions for improving adherence to medication prescribed for the primary prevention of cardiovascular disease in adults. *Cochrane Database Syst. Rev.* **2017**, *2017*. [CrossRef]
41. Hamine, S.; Gerth-Guyette, E.; Faulx, D.; Green, B.B.; Ginsburg, A.S. Impact of mhealth chronic disease management on treatment adherence and patient outcomes: A systematic review. *J. Med. Internet Res.* **2015**, *17*, e3951. [CrossRef]
42. Kebapci, A.; Ozkaynak, M.; Lareau, S.C. Effects of Ehealth-based interventions on adherence to components of cardiac rehabilitation: A systematic review. *J. Cardiovasc. Nurs.* **2020**, *35*, 74–85. [CrossRef]
43. Rathbone, A.L.; Prescott, J. The use of mobile apps and sms messaging as physical and mental health interventions: Systematic review. *J. Med. Internet Res.* **2017**, *19*, e7740. [CrossRef]
44. Firth, J.; Torous, J.; Nicholas, J.; Carney, R.; Pratap, A.; Rosenbaum, S.; Sarris, J. The efficacy of smartphone-based mental health interventions for depressive symptoms: A meta-analysis of randomized controlled trials. *World Psychiatry* **2017**, *16*, 287–298. [CrossRef]
45. Leahy, R.L.; Tirch, D.; Napolitano, L.A. *Emotion Regulation in Psychotherapy: A Practitioner's Guide*; Guilford Press: New York, NY, USA, 2011; ISBN 978-1-4625-0237-0.
46. Zigmond, A.S.; Snaith, R.P. The hospital anxiety and depression scale. *Acta Psychiatr. Scand.* **1983**, *67*, 361–370. [CrossRef]
47. Terol, M.C.; López-Roig, S.; Rodríguez-Marín, J.; Martín-Aragón, M.; Pastor, M.A.; Reig, M.T. Propiedades psicométricas de la escala Hospitalaria de Ansiedad y Depresión (HAD) en población española. [Hospital Anxiety and Depression Scale (HAD): Psychometric Properties in Spanish Population.]. *Ansiedad Estrés* **2007**, *13*, 163–176.
48. Caprara, G.V.; Alessandri, G.; Eisenberg, N.; Kupfer, A.; Steca, P.; Caprara, M.G.; Yamaguchi, S.; Fukuzawa, A.; Abela, J. The positivity scale. *Psychol. Assess.* **2012**, *24*, 701–712. [CrossRef]
49. Watson, D.; Clark, L.A.; Tellegen, A. Development and validation of brief measures of positive and negative affect: The PANAS scales. *J. Pers. Soc. Psychol.* **1988**, *54*, 1063–1070. [CrossRef]
50. Tabernero, C.; Chambel, M.J.; Curral, L.; Arana, J.M. The role of task-oriented versus relationshiporiented leadership on normative contract and group performance. *Soc. Behav. Personal.* **2009**, *37*, 1391–1404. [CrossRef]
51. Ritter, P.L.; Lorig, K. The english and spanish self-efficacy to manage chronic disease scale measures were validated using multiple studies. *J. Clin. Epidemiol.* **2014**, *67*, 1265–1273. [CrossRef]
52. Steca, P.; Greco, A.; Cappelletti, E.; Monzani, D.; Pancani, L.; Ferrari, G.; Politi, A.; Gestra, R.; Malfatto, G.; Parati, G.; et al. Cardiovascular management self-efficacy: Psychometric properties of a new scale and its usefulness in a rehabilitation context. *Ann. Behav. Med.* **2015**, *49*, 660–674. [CrossRef]
53. Faul, F.; Erdfelder, E.; Buchner, A.; Lang, A.-G. Statistical power analyses using G*Power 3.1: Tests for correlation and regression analyses. *Behav. Res. Methods* **2009**, *41*, 1149–1160. [CrossRef]
54. Huffman, J.C.; Feig, E.H.; Millstein, R.A.; Freedman, M.; Healy, B.C.; Chung, W.-J.; Amonoo, H.L.; Malloy, L.; Slawsby, E.; Januzzi, J.L.; et al. Usefulness of a positive psychology-motivational interviewing intervention to promote positive affect and physical activity after an acute coronary syndrome. *Am. J. Cardiol.* **2019**, *123*, 1906–1914. [CrossRef]
55. Meyerowitz-Katz, G.; Ravi, S.; Arnolda, L.; Feng, X.; Maberly, G.; Astell-Burt, T. Rates of attrition and dropout in app-based interventions for chronic disease: Systematic review and meta-analysis. *J. Med. Internet Res.* **2020**, *22*, e20283. [CrossRef]
56. Gao, Z.; Chen, Z.; Sun, A.; Deng, X. Gender differences in cardiovascular disease. *Med. Nov. Technol. Devices* **2019**, *4*, 100025. [CrossRef]
57. Appleton, A.A.; Buka, S.L.; Loucks, E.B.; Gilman, S.E.; Kubzansky, L.D. Divergent associations of adaptive and maladaptive emotion regulation strategies with inflammation. *Health Psychol.* **2013**, *32*, 748–756. [CrossRef]
58. Gross, J.J.; John, O.P. Individual differences in two emotion regulation processes: Implications for affect, relationships, and well-being. *J. Pers. Soc. Psychol.* **2003**, *85*, 348–362. [CrossRef]
59. Kubzansky, L.D.; Park, N.; Peterson, C.; Vokonas, P.; Sparrow, D. Healthy psychological functioning and incident coronary heart disease: The importance of self-regulation. *Arch. Gen. Psychiatry* **2011**, *68*, 400–408. [CrossRef]
60. Charlson, M.E.; Wells, M.T.; Peterson, J.C.; Boutin-Foster, C.; Ogedegbe, G.O.; Mancuso, C.A.; Hollenberg, J.P.; Allegrante, J.P.; Jobe, J.; Isen, A.M. Mediators and moderators of behavior change in patients with chronic cardiopulmonary disease: The impact of positive affect and self-affirmation. *Transl. Behav. Med.* **2014**, *4*, 7–17. [CrossRef]
61. Nsamenang, S.A.; Hirsch, J.K. Positive psychological determinants of treatment adherence among primary care patients. *Prim. Health Care Res. Dev.* **2015**, *16*, 398–406. [CrossRef]

62. Hoen, P.W.; Denollet, J.; De Jonge, P.; Whooley, M.A. Positive affect and survival in patients with stable coronary heart disease: Findings from the heart and soul study. *J. Clin. Psychiatry* **2013**, *74*, 14722. [CrossRef]
63. DuBois, C.M.; Lopez, O.V.; Beale, E.E.; Healy, B.C.; Boehm, J.K.; Huffman, J.C. Relationships between positive psychological constructs and health outcomes in patients with cardiovascular disease: A systematic review. *Int. J. Cardiol.* **2015**, *195*, 265–280. [CrossRef]
64. Tabernero, C.; Gutiérrez-Domingo, T.; Vecchione, M.; Cuadrado, E.; Castillo-Mayén, R.; Rubio, S.; Arenas, A.; Delgado-Lista, J.; Pérez-Martínez, P.; Luque, B. Correction: A longitudinal study on perceived health in cardiovascular patients: The role of conscientiousness, subjective wellbeing and cardiac self-efficacy. *PLoS ONE* **2020**, *15*, e0229582. [CrossRef]
65. Gomis-Pastor, M.; Mirabet Perez, S.; Roig Minguell, E.; Brossa Loidi, V.; Lopez Lopez, L.; Ros Abarca, S.; Galvez Tugas, E.; Mas-Malagarriga, N.; Mangues Bafalluy, M.A. Mobile health to improve adherence and patient experience in heart transplantation recipients: The MHeart trial. *Healthcare* **2021**, *9*, 463. [CrossRef]
66. Mohammadi, N.; Aghayousefi, A.; Nikrahan, G.R.; Adams, C.N.; Alipour, A.; Sadeghi, M.; Roohafza, H.; Celano, C.M.; Huffman, J.C. A Randomized trial of an optimism training intervention in patients with heart disease. *Gen. Hosp. Psychiatry* **2018**, *51*, 46–53. [CrossRef]
67. Nikrahan, G.R.; Eshaghi, L.; Massey, C.N.; Hemmat, A.; Amonoo, H.L.; Healy, B.; Huffman, J.C. Randomized controlled trial of a well-being intervention in cardiac patients. *Gen. Hosp. Psychiatry* **2019**, *61*, 116–124. [CrossRef]
68. Samayoa, L.; Grace, S.L.; Gravely, S.; Scott, L.B.; Marzolini, S.; Colella, T.J.F. Sex differences in cardiac rehabilitation enrollment: A meta-analysis. *Can. J. Cardiol.* **2014**, *30*, 793–800. [CrossRef]
69. Resurrección, D.M.; Motrico, E.; Rigabert, A.; Rubio-Valera, M.; Conejo-Cerón, S.; Pastor, L.; Moreno-Peral, P. Barriers for nonparticipation and dropout of women in cardiac rehabilitation programs: A systematic review. *J. Womens Health 2002* **2017**, *26*, 849–859. [CrossRef]

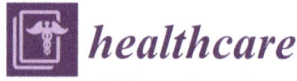

Review

Patient Satisfaction with Telemedicine in Adults with Diabetes: A Systematic Review

Hidetaka Hamasaki

Hamasaki Clinic, 2-21-4 Kagoshima, Kagoshima 890-0046, Japan; h-hamasaki@umin.ac.jp; Tel.: +81-99-2503535; Fax: +81-99-2501470

Abstract: Patient satisfaction assessment is essential for improving the quality of healthcare. Diabetes management using telemedicine technology is promising in the 21st century. However, the number of randomised controlled trials (RCTs) examining the effect of telemedicine on satisfaction in patients with diabetes is limited. This systematic review aimed to summarise the current evidence on patient satisfaction with telemedicine in adults with diabetes and discuss related issues and future directions of telemedicine in patients with diabetes. The author systematically searched PubMed/MEDLINE, Embase and The Cochrane Library, and a total of six RCTs were eligible for this review. Patient satisfaction with telemedicine was as high as conventional face-to-face care; however, telemedicine appeared not to significantly increase patient satisfaction compared with conventional face-to-face care in the included studies. Significant heterogeneity was noted between the studies, including participants' age, study duration, the method of assessing patient satisfaction and types of telemedicine. Further studies are required to provide firm evidence to healthcare providers who are willing to use telemedicine in diabetes management. Telemedicine technology has been advancing and is a key tool in providing high-quality healthcare to patients with diabetes in the 21st century.

Keywords: patient satisfaction; telemedicine; information technology; digital health; type 1 diabetes; type 2 diabetes

Citation: Hamasaki, H. Patient Satisfaction with Telemedicine in Adults with Diabetes: A Systematic Review. *Healthcare* **2022**, *10*, 1677. https://doi.org/10.3390/healthcare10091677

Academic Editor: Daniele Giansanti

Received: 7 August 2022
Accepted: 1 September 2022
Published: 2 September 2022

Publisher's Note: MDPI stays neutral with regard to jurisdictional claims in published maps and institutional affiliations.

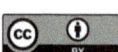

Copyright: © 2022 by the author. Licensee MDPI, Basel, Switzerland. This article is an open access article distributed under the terms and conditions of the Creative Commons Attribution (CC BY) license (https://creativecommons.org/licenses/by/4.0/).

1. Introduction

Information technology has rapidly advanced since the Internet was developed and became widely used in the 1990s [1]. In healthcare, information technology has been expanding in applying electronic medical records [2], performing big data analytics [3] and utilising artificial intelligence for the diagnosis and treatment of various diseases [4], which is changing the conventional medical practice. Diabetes is a chronic disease that is significantly influenced by diet, physical activity, behaviour and medication adherence in daily life; therefore, interactive communication between healthcare providers and patients via telemedicine technology is suitable for managing patients with diabetes [5]. Indeed, the use of telemedicine was effective for glycaemic control with a mean difference of haemoglobin A1c (HbA1c) of −0.415% (95% confidence interval [CI], −0.482% to −0.348%) in patients with type 2 diabetes [6] and −0.18% (95% CI, −0.04% to −0.33%) in patients with type 1 diabetes [7], and cost-effective for diabetic retinopathy screening [8]. Moreover, the implementation of telemedicine using a high-speed network system and wearable devices was an effective measure for patient care and was accepted by both clinicians and patients with high satisfaction during the coronavirus disease 2019 (COVID-19) pandemic [9,10]. Telemedicine is a promising approach for improving the quality of healthcare [11] as well as health outcomes of patients [12] and reducing operational costs of healthcare services [8] in the management of diabetes; thus, this technology will be essential to provide healthcare effectively and safely to patients with diabetes in the 21st century. The next pandemic could occur sooner than we think, and in-person healthcare may not be allowed in such a circumstance. Conversely, the effect of telemedicine on satisfaction in patients with diabetes is not fully investigated. Kruse et al. [13] examined the association between telemedicine and patient satisfaction by analysing 44 published articles and found that patient satisfaction was associated with some factors of telemedicine, including outcomes, ease of use, communication and travel time. However, the study design of the included studies was not limited to randomised controlled trials (RCTs), and only four studies were noted in which study participants were patients with diabetes. Pascoe [14] stated that patient satisfaction assessment is critical for understanding the function of the healthcare system. Moreover, patients with high satisfaction are likely to have high medication adherence, leading to improved health outcomes [15].

Hence, assessing patient satisfaction with telemedicine in diabetes management is crucial. The author developed the following research question: In patients with diabetes (P), what is the effect of telemedicine (I) on patient satisfaction (O) compared with conventional care (C)? This study aims to investigate the effect of telemedicine on patient satisfaction in patients with diabetes.

2. Materials and Methods

This systematic review was conducted following the Preferred Reporting Items for Systematic Reviews and Meta-Analyses guidelines [16] (Supplementary File).

2.1. Search Strategy

The author searched PubMed/MEDLINE, Embase and The Cochrane Library from their inception to June 2022. The author used Medical Subject Headings (MeSH) terms 'telemedicine' AND 'diabetes mellitus' AND 'patient satisfaction' for the systematic search. Based on the National Institute of Health's definition of telemedicine [17] and the study by Sood et al. [18], telemedicine is defined as the use of communication technologies for delivery of healthcare services at a distance, which involves virtual visits between physicians and patients and remote monitoring. Telemedicine is broadly defined as the use of various communication modalities [17]. There could be some studies that refer to a specific communication modality alone. Therefore, the author also used the search terms 'virtual visit' OR 'digital health' OR 'remote monitoring' OR 'mHealth' OR 'eHealth' as a substitute for the MeSH term 'telemedicine'. The author included articles in English that were published in peer-reviewed journals.

2.2. Inclusion and Exclusion Criteria

The articles had to meet the following criteria: (1) the study design had to be RCT, (2) the study population had to be adults with types 2 or 1 diabetes, (3) the intervention had to be telemedicine implementation or telemedicine in addition to conventional in-person care and (4) the study had to report a pre- and post-satisfaction score. Reviews, observational studies, case reports, editorials, letters, conference papers and study protocols were excluded. Qualitative studies without quantitative analysis for patient satisfaction were excluded. Studies that reported patient satisfaction in the intervention group alone were also excluded.

2.3. Study Quality Assessment

The revised Cochrane risk-of-bias tool for randomised trials was used for quality assessment in the included studies [19]. The assessment was categorised into one of the following three levels: 'high risk of bias', 'some concerns' and 'low risk of bias' based on risk-of-bias tools [20].

3. Results

3.1. Study Selection

The systematic literature search yielded 5852 articles. Of these, 547 RCTs were identified. Moreover, 60 studies that investigated the effect of telemedicine on patient satisfaction in patients with diabetes were fully reviewed to determine their relevance. Six articles were eligible for this systematic review. The flow of the systematic search process is depicted in Figure 1.

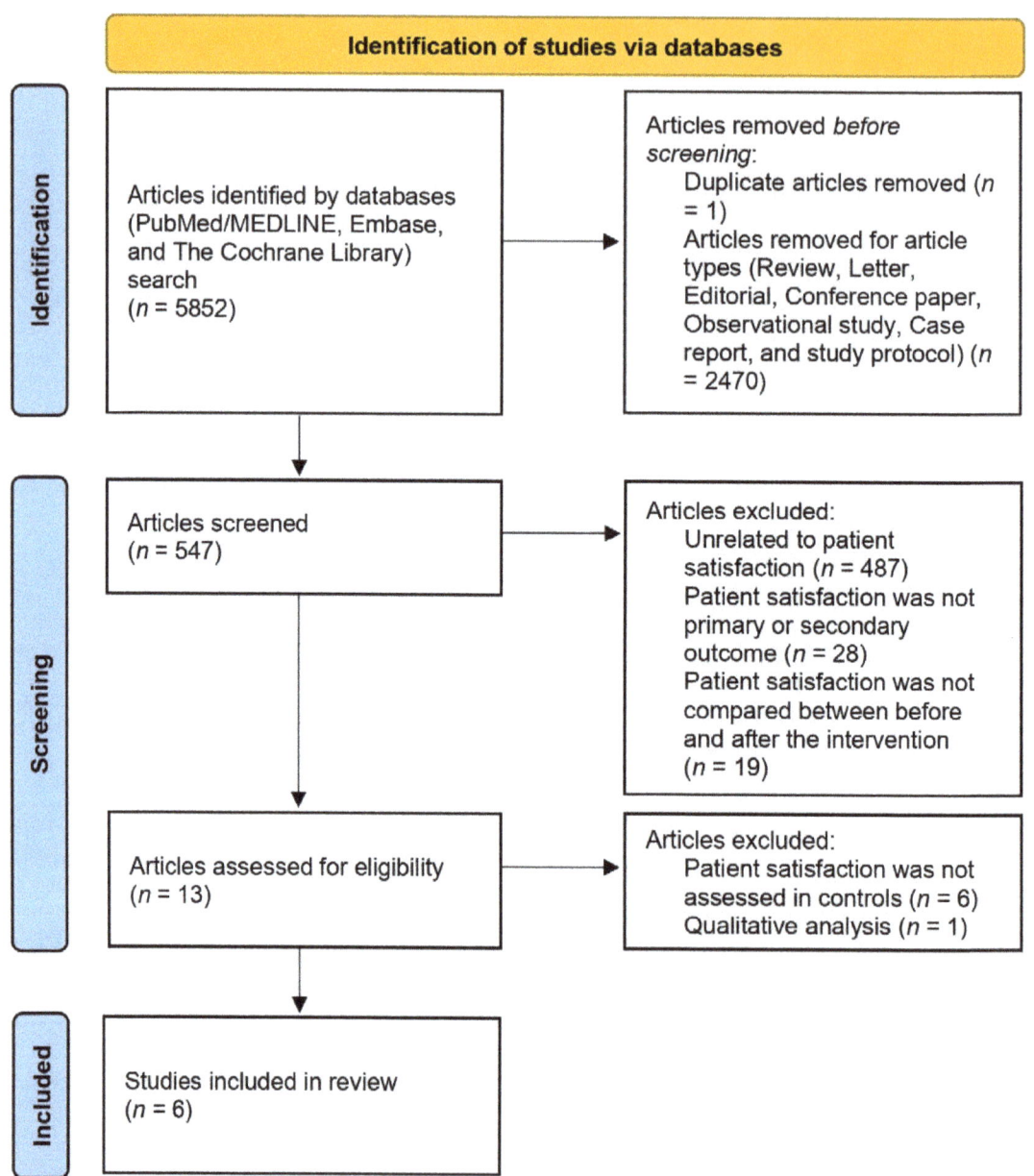

Figure 1. PRISMA flow diagram.

3.2. Study Characteristics

The characteristics of the included studies are summarised in Table 1.

Izquierdo et al. [21] investigated the hypothesis that diabetes education via telemedicine was as effective as in-person for the management of patients with diabetes. Patients in the intervention group had three diabetes education visits via teleconferencing, whereas patients in the control group had one-on-one in-person visits. The first visit included 1-h consultations with a diabetes specialist nurse and dietitian. The second and third visits were 30-min consultations at 4–6 and 8–12 weeks, respectively. Physicians in charge were unaware whether the patient was allocated to the intervention or control group. Of the study participants, 88% completed the three diabetes education visits and their changes in glycaemic control and satisfaction were analysed. Although glycaemic control measured by HbA1c levels and patient satisfaction in patients who received telemedicine were not superior to those in patients who received conventional in-person care, telemedicine was as effective as in-person care for treating diabetes, and patient satisfaction was similarly high in both groups. The treatment satisfaction measured by the Diabetes Treatment Satisfaction Questionnaire (DTSQ) (a maximum total score of 36) increased from 22.8 ± 8.6 to 31.3 ± 4.2 in the intervention group ($p < 0.001$). Furthermore, the authors administered the Telemedicine Patient Satisfaction Survey [22] in the intervention group at the 3-month visit and found that overall satisfaction was relatively high (4.3 ± 1.3 on a scale of 1–5) and 84% of the participants wanted to continue telemedicine. The authors concluded that diabetes education via telemedicine would provide an opportunity for patients with diabetes who could not acquire high-quality care due to underserved areas and help motivate and empower them to improve health-related behaviours.

Yaron et al. [23] examined the effectiveness, safety, acceptability and cost-effectiveness of telemedicine in patients with type 1 diabetes using insulin pumps. Patients in the intervention group downloaded blood glucose data from their insulin pumps once a month and transferred the information to the clinic using a web application. Physicians reviewed the data and sent recommendations immediately on adjusting insulin doses and support messages to maintain and improve motivation. Additionally, study participants had face-to-face visits once at 6-month intervals, totalling three visits during the study period. Conversely, patients in the control group had face-to-face visits only at 3-month intervals, totalling five visits during the study period. Patient satisfaction with the diabetes treatment was high in both groups: the satisfaction scores were 1.8 ± 1.24 and 1.4 ± 1.3 in the intervention and control groups, respectively (scores ranged from +3 'much more satisfied now' to −3 'much less satisfied now'). Furthermore, patients in the intervention group were more satisfied with continuing the telemedicine than those who received standard care (2.1 ± 1.21 vs. 1.4 ± 1.35, $p = 0.04$). Although the improvement in glycaemic control was not statistically significant, the frequency of hypo- and hyperglycaemic events did not differ between groups, and the direct and indirect total costs of care were reduced by 24% and 22%, respectively, in patients receiving telemedicine; hence, the telemedicine approach was highly satisfactory, safe and cost-effective in the management of patients with type 1 diabetes.

Cho et al. [24] considered the barrier that older adults could not use manual Internet-based telemedicine successfully and investigated the efficacy and feasibility of an Internet-integrated device, which automatically uploads patient data for diabetes management. The blood glucose and blood pressure data of the study participants were automatically uploaded to the online server using the health gateway device. Study participants could also communicate with the healthcare providers about their weight, diet, exercise, hypoglycaemic events and any other questions through the device and received personal recommendations every week (for the first 3 months) or every other week (for the last 3 months). The total DTSQ score was not significantly increased from 25.0 ± 6.3 at baseline to 27.9 ± 6.48 at the end of the study in the intervention group as well as that of the control group (25.9 ± 5.9–26.7 ± 5.8). However, the total DTSQ score was significantly higher in the intervention group than that in the control group at the end of the study ($p < 0.05$). Additionally, HbA1c levels and waist circumference were decreased more in the intervention group than those in the control group. No significant difference in adverse events between groups was reported. The authors did not discuss patient satisfaction in the discussion section; however, high patient satisfaction was the result of improved glycaemic control rather than telemedicine itself.

Kirwan et al. [25] investigated the effectiveness of a freely available smartphone application on the management of patients with type 1 diabetes. Patients in the intervention group were instructed to use a smartphone application that allows users to enter data regarding diabetes self-management, such as diet, physical activity, blood glucose, insulin doses and other medications in addition to usual care (face-to-face visit every 3 months). They also received personalised feedback from a certified diabetes educator to improve diabetes management at least once a week during the first six months. The mean score of 'Satisfaction' in the Diabetes Quality of Life (DQOL) questionnaire was increased both in the intervention and control groups (3.20 ± 0.66–3.42 ± 0.68 and 3.09 ± 0.55–3.29 ± 0.65, respectively); however, this finding was not statistically significant, and no difference between groups was observed. Glycaemic control measured by HbA1c levels was significantly improved in the intervention group compared with that in the control group. This result suggests that patient satisfaction was not associated with improving glycaemic control. The authors pointed out that the level of engagement of study participants in telemedicine studies seemed to be underreported [26]. Even if evidence was noted of its effectiveness in clinical study settings, telemedicine without in-person communication between patients and healthcare providers may not frequently be practical for diabetes self-management in the real world.

Ruiz de Adana et al. [27] examined the impact of telemedicine on glycaemic control; health-related quality of life, including patient satisfaction with treatment; physicians' satisfaction in patients with type 1 diabetes. Patients in the control group were followed up by face-to-face visits every 3 months, whereas those in the intervention group performed the second visit remotely using an Internet-based telemedicine system that helps patients make decisions on diabetes management. Patients in the intervention group could check the information on self-monitored blood glucose values, insulin doses, carbohydrate consumption, physical activity and other health-related data. HbA1c levels, the number of hypoglycaemia episodes and indices of glycaemic variability did not differ between groups at the end of the study. The satisfaction score with treatment increased in the control group and slightly decreased in the intervention group; however, no significant difference between groups was observed at the end of the study. Conversely, physicians' satisfaction score with the telemedicine system was 6.28 (on a scale of 0–10). The authors stated that the clinical efficacy and safety of the telemedicine system were similar to conventional face-to-face visits. Thus, some face-to-face visits could be replaced by telemedicine, which would result in improving access to healthcare in cases with low medical resources.

Sood et al. [28] conducted a cluster-RCT to compare HbA1c, blood pressure, lipid profile and patient satisfaction measured by DTSQ between patients who had telemedicine consultations via videoconference once a week and those who had usual face-to-face consultations at the diabetes clinic. HbA1c levels were decreased in both groups; however, no statistically significant difference between groups was noted. The DTSQ score changed from 24.1 ± 0.8 to 23.8 ± 7.3 in the intervention group and from 23.8 ± 7.3 to 24.0 ± 7.7 in the control group, respectively. The change in the DTSQ score did not differ between groups. However, more patients in the intervention group were highly satisfied with the visit than those in the control group (61.2% vs. 40.8%, $p = 0.004$). Furthermore, more patients in the intervention group answered that specialists understood the patient's situation (97.0% vs. 88.4%, $p = 0.009$) and were comfortable with the number of providers during the visit (83.0% vs. 72.3%, $p < 0.001$), and fewer patients in the intervention group answered on the disagreement of the benefit of the visits (2.4% vs. 14.1%, $p < 0.001$) than those in the control group. More than 99% of the participants agreed that telemedicine improved accessibility to medical care. These results indicated that telemedicine was as effective as usual care for managing diabetes and patient experience with telemedicine was highly appreciated.

Table 1. Summary of included studies.

Reference	Country	Study Design	Study Period	Subjects	Study Outcomes	Intervention Control Telemedicine Tool	Results (Patient Satisfaction)
Izquierdo et al. (2003) [21]	USA	Randomised, controlled, parallel-group trial	3 months	56 adults with diabetes, 10 dropouts Intervention group (thirteen men and nine women): Age: 61.37 ± 8.95 years, BMI: 31.34 ± 6.20 kg/m^2, HbA1c: 8.33 ± 1.63% Control group (eight men and sixteen women): Age: 53.95 ± 10.08 years, BMI: 35.95 ± 9.22 kg/m^2, HbA1c: 8.68 ± 2.17%	Primary: HbA1c Secondary: Weight, BMI, PAID scale, DQOL score, ADS score, DTSQ score, Treatment satisfaction	Telemedicine (videoconference)/in-person Real-time one-on-one teleconferencing using a private ISDN line.	Patient satisfaction ↑ (DTSQ score: 22.8 ± 8.6 to 31.3 ± 4.2, $p < 0.001$ in the intervention group; 23.8 ± 7.9 to 29.1 ± 5.3, $p < 0.001$ in the control group). No difference in satisfaction scores between groups. No interaction of group by time.
Yaron et al. (2019) [23]	Israel	Randomised, controlled, parallel-group trial	12 months	74 patients with type 1 diabetes on insulin pumps, seven dropouts Intervention group (19 men and 12 women): Age: 43 ± 11 years, BMI: 26.6 ± 4.6 kg/m^2, HbA1c: 7.59 ± 0.82% Control group (13 men and 23 women): Age: 45 ± 14 years, BMI: 25.5 ± 3.8 kg/m^2, HbA1c: 7.95 ± 0.6%	Primary: HbA1c Secondary: QoL score (ADDQoL score), DTSQ score, changes in total hypoglycaemic events (blood glucose ≤ 70 mg/dL) and hyperglycaemic events (blood glucose ≥ 300 mg/dL), cost-effectiveness of telemedicine	Telemedicine (Carelink Pro Software)/Face-to-face visit Data from the insulin pump and glucometer are transmitted to the clinic by Carelink Pro Software. Physicians review the data and document the recommendations.	Patient satisfaction ↑ DTSQ score of Q8 'willingness to continue' was higher in the intervention group than that in the control group (2.1 vs. 1.4, $p = 0.04$). QoL. →

Table 1. Cont.

Reference	Country	Study Design	Study Period	Subjects	Study Outcomes	Intervention Control Telemedicine Tool	Results (Patient Satisfaction)
Cho et al. (2017) [24]	South Korea	Randomised, controlled, parallel-group trial	6 months	484 patients with type 2 diabetes. Intervention group (152 men and 88 women): Age: 53.4 ± 8.7 years, BMI: 25.5 ± 3.2 kg/m^2, HbA1c: 7.81 ± 0.66%. Control group (155 men and 89 women): Age: 52.9 ± 9.2 years, BMI: 25.6 ± 3.4 kg/m^2, HbA1c: 7.86 ± 0.89%	Primary: HbA1c, glycaemic control Secondary: Anthropometric and biochemical parameters, SF-12 score, DTSQ score, adverse events of telemedicine	Internet-based communication (Hi-Care)/Outpatient clinic visit. Patients upload the glucose and blood pressure data automatically to the online server using the device. Patients can see recommendation messages from the medical team on the device.	Patient satisfaction ↑ (DTSQ score: 25.0 ± 6.3 to 27.9 ± 6.48, NS in the intervention group; 25.9 ± 5.9 to 26.7 ± 5.8, NS in the control group). DTSQ score was significantly higher in the intervention group than that in the control group 6 months after the intervention (27.9 ± 6.48 vs. 26.7 ± 5.8, $p < 0.05$). QoL →
Kirwan et al. (2013) [25]	Australia	Randomised, controlled, parallel-group trial	9 months	72 adults with type 1 diabetes, 19 dropouts. Intervention group (19 men and 17 women): Age: 35.97 ± 10.67 years, BMI: No description, HbA1c: 9.08 ± 1.18%. Control group (nine men and twenty-seven women): Age: 34.42 ± 10.26 years, BMI: No description, HbA1c: 8.47 ± 0.86%	Primary: HbA1c Secondary: DES-SF score, SDSCA score, DQOL score	Smartphone application (Glucose Buddy)/Usual care. Freely available iPhone application that allows patients to manually enter diet, physical activity, blood glucose levels, insulin dosages and other medications. The application data were reviewed by a certified diabetes educator via a web interface.	Patient satisfaction → (DQOL score 'Satisfaction': 3.20 ± 0.66 to 3.42 ± 0.68, NS in the intervention group; 3.09 ± 0.55 to 3.29 ± 0.65, NS in the control group). No difference in satisfaction scores between groups. No interaction of group by time. No change in either group in relation to self-efficacy, self-care activities and QoL.

Table 1. *Cont.*

Reference	Country	Study Design	Study Period	Subjects	Study Outcomes	Intervention Control Telemedicine Tool	Results (Patient Satisfaction)
						Telemedicine (Diabetic) + face-to-face visit/Face-to-face visit	
Ruiz de Adana et al. (2020) [27]	Spain	Randomised, controlled, parallel-group trial	6 months	388 patients with type 1 diabetes, 58 dropouts Intervention group (90 men and 73 women): Age: 33.78 ± 9.77 years, BMI: 26.0 ± 4.6 kg/m^2, HbA1c: 66 participants <7% Control group (94 men and 73 women): Age: 36.22 ± 10.78 years, BMI: 26.0 ± 4.6 kg/m^2, HbA1c: 68 participants <7%	Primary: Mean change of HbA1c Secondary: Mean blood glucose, glycaemic variability, DQOL score, DDS score, FH-15 score	Internet-based telemedicine system (web- and mobile-based) designed for monitoring patients with diabetes. Patients can download their self-monitored blood glucose data and include information regarding carbohydrate consumption, physical activity, insulin dosages and other health data. Physicians can review the data and evaluate metabolic control statistics or treatment reports.	Patient satisfaction → (DQOL score 'Satisfaction': 72.0 ± 12.4 to 71.7 ± 14.8, NS in the intervention group; 67.8 ± 16.1 to 69.5 ± 16.3, NS in the control group). The satisfaction score (satisfaction) was higher in the intervention group than that in the control group (72.0 vs. 67.8 $p < 0.05$) at the first visit; however, no difference in satisfaction between groups was observed at the end of study.

Table 1. Cont.

Reference	Country	Study Design	Study Period	Subjects	Study Outcomes	Intervention Telemedicine Tool	Control	Results (Patient Satisfaction)
Sood et al. (2018) [28]	USA	Cluster-randomised, controlled, trial	18 months	282 patients with diabetes Intervention group (one hundred ninety-eight men and one woman): Age: 61.6 ± 9.4 years, BMI: No description, HbA1c: 10.0 ± 1.6% Control group (83 men): Age: 61.1 ± 10.0 years, BMI: No description, HbA1c: 9.4 ± 2.1%	Primary: HbA1c Secondary: Medication use, blood pressure, low-density lipoprotein cholesterol, high-density lipoprotein cholesterol, triglycerides, DTSQ score	Telemedicine (videoconference)/Usual care Telemedicine consultation via videoconference at the community-based outpatient clinic accompanied by one healthcare provider. The medical team interviews and advises the patient to manage diabetes effectively.		Patient satisfaction → (DTSQ score: 24.1 ± 8.0 to 23.8 ± 7.3, NS in the intervention group; 23.8 ± 7.3 to 24.0 ± 7.7, NS in the control group). No difference in satisfaction scores between groups. However, the proportion of patients who were very satisfied with the consultation was higher in the intervention group than that in the control group (61.2% vs. 40.8%, $p = 0.004$).

↑ Increase, → no change, *BMI* body mass index, *HbA1c* haemoglobin A1c, *PAID* Problem Areas in Diabetes, *DQOL* Diabetes Quality of Life, *ADS* Appraisal of Diabetes Scale, *DTSQ* Diabetes Treatment Satisfaction Questionnaire, *ISDN* integrated services digital network, *QoL* quality of life, *ADDQoL* Audit of Diabetes Quality of Life, *NS* not significant, *SF-12* 12-item Short Form Survey, *DES-SF* Diabetes Empowerment Scale-Short Form, *SDSCA* Summary of Diabetes Self-Care Activities, *DDS* Diabetes Distress Scale, *FH-15* Fear of Hypoglycaemia scale.

Tables 2 and 3 visually summarise the relationship of patient satisfaction with glycaemic control (changes in HbA1c levels) (Table 2) and telemedicine modalities (Table 3). There was no significant relationship of patient satisfaction with glycaemic control and a specific telemedicine modality.

Table 2. The relationship between patient satisfaction and glycaemic control.

Study	Glycaemic Control (HbA1c)	Patient Satisfaction
Izquierdo et al. [21]	↓	↑
Cho et al. [24]		
Yaron et al. [23]	→	↑
Kirwan et al. [25]	↓	→
Ruiz de Adana et al. [27]	→	→
Sood et al. [28]		

↑ Increase, → no change, ↓ decrease, *HbA1c* haemoglobin A1c.

Table 3. The relationship between patient satisfaction and telemedicine modalities.

Study	Telemedicine Modalities	Patient Satisfaction
Izquierdo et al. [21]	Virtual visit	↑
Sood et al. [28]		→
Cho et al. [24]		↑
Yaron et al. [23]	Remote monitoring	↑
Kirwan et al. [25]		→
Ruiz de Adana et al. [27]	Virtual visit + Remote monitoring	→

↑ Increase, → no change, ↓ decrease.

3.3. Study Quality

The overall risk of bias was 'high' except for the study by Yaron et al. [23] (Figure 2).

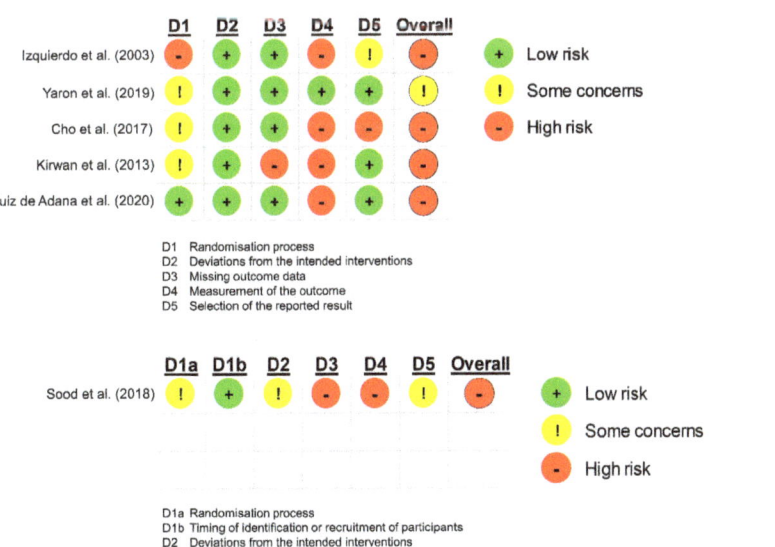

Figure 2. Risk of bias in the included studies. This figure was automatically made by RoB2 tool: https://www.riskofbias.info/welcome/rob-2-0-tool/current-version-of-rob-2 (accessed on 1 January 2022).

Most studies involved some concerns in the random sequence process, and the studies by Izquierdo et al. [21], Kirwan et al. [25] and Sood et al. [28] had some differences in participant characteristics between the intervention and control groups at baseline. The most critical factor for the high risk of bias in the included studies is the open-label design, except for the study by Yaron et al. [23] (single-blinded). Therefore, the outcome measurements may have been influenced by researcher biases.

4. Discussion

This systematic review demonstrated that patient satisfaction was high in patients receiving telemedicine. However, most of the included studies reported no significant difference in patient satisfaction between the telemedicine and usual (face-to-face) care groups. The study by Cho et al. [24] showed that telemedicine significantly increased patient satisfaction compared with face-to-face visits; however, this result may have been influenced by the course of treatment for diabetes because the study participants were not blinded and were aware about how their glycaemic control changed during the study period. In contrast, Ruiz de Adana et al. [27] indicated that patient satisfaction could decrease with the implementation of telemedicine; however, patients in the intervention group used telemedicine in only one of three visits, which suggests that the effect of telemedicine alone on patient satisfaction was not sufficiently evaluated.

Significant heterogeneity was observed between the included studies, such as participants' age, study duration and the method of assessing patient satisfaction. However, the telemedicine tool used in previous studies varied. The article by Izquierdo et al. [21] was published in 2003; thus, data transmission speed via the Internet was limited. The study participants communicated with each other using Integrated Services Digital Network (128 Kb/s) in real-time, which is much slower than the current Fifth Generation Mobile Communication System (5G), whose theoretical data transmission speed is ~10–30 Gb/s [29]. No specific telemedicine device/application was used in this study. Similarly, Yaron et al. [23] and Sood et al. [28] did not use a specific device/application (Yaron et al. used software that enabled reviewing patients' data from the insulin pump and glucometer). In contrast, Cho et al. [26] used a health gateway system (HiCare) with Internet-based communication, Kirwan et al. [25] used a smartphone application and Ruiz de Adana et al. [27] used a remote monitoring system that allowed access to patients' data from smartphones. Each system or application has different functionality and usability for the management of diabetes; hence, it may be challenging to assess patient satisfaction with 'telemedicine' as a whole concept.

The sufficient validity and reliability of the patient satisfaction questionnaire are essential for patient satisfaction surveys. For example, the Telemedicine Patient Satisfaction Survey [22] used in the study by Izquierdo et al. [21] is an established approach to assess patient satisfaction, which was extensively tested in previous studies [30,31]; however, according to Hajesmaeel-Gohari and Bahaadinbeigy [32], this questionnaire is not frequently used these days.

In contrast, DTSQ is widely used for evaluating patient satisfaction with the treatment of diabetes [33]. Four of six studies in this systematic review used DTSQ to assess patient satisfaction. DTSQ consists of eight question items that are rated on a seven-point Likert scale (ranging from zero to six): Q1 'How satisfied are you with your current treatment?', Q2 'How often have you felt that your blood sugars have been unacceptably high recently?', Q3 'How often have you felt that your blood sugars have been unacceptably low recently?', Q4 'How convenient have you been finding your treatment to be recently?', Q5 'How flexible have you been finding your treatment to be recently?', Q6 'How satisfied are you with your understanding of your diabetes?', Q7 'Would you recommend this form of treatment to someone else with your kind of diabetes?' and Q8 'How satisfied would you be to continue with your present form of treatment?' [34]. Considering that this questionnaire aims to assess patient satisfaction in terms of diabetes treatment, that is, diet, exercise, type and dose of oral hypoglycaemic agents and insulin injections, it should be noted that satisfaction with the healthcare delivery system may not be adequately evaluated. Conversely, the other two studies used the DQOL questionnaire to evaluate patient satisfaction. The DQOL questionnaire has the following four sections: 'Satisfaction', 'Impact', 'Worry: Social/Vocational' and 'Worry: Diabetes Related'. The Satisfaction section consists of the following 15 items that are rated on a five-point Likert scale (ranging from one to five): Q1 'How satisfied are you with the amount of time it takes to manage your diabetes?', Q2 'How satisfied are you with the amount of time you spend getting checkups?', Q3 'How satisfied are you with the time it takes to determine your sugar level?', Q4 'How satisfied are you with your current treatment?', Q5 'How satisfied are you with the flexibility you have in your diet?', Q6 'How satisfied are you with the burden your diabetes is placing on your family?', Q7 'How satisfied are you with your knowledge about your diabetes?', Q8 'How satisfied are you with your sleep?', Q9 'How satisfied are you with your social relationships and friendships?', Q10 'How satisfied are you with your sex life?', Q11 'How satisfied are you with your work, school, and household activities?', Q12 'How satisfied are you with the appearance of your body?', Q13 'How satisfied are you with the time you spend exercising?', Q14 'How satisfied are you with your leisure time?' and Q15 'How satisfied are you with life in general?' [35]. The Satisfaction section of the DQOL questionnaire is designed to assess satisfaction with not diabetes management but a patient's whole life; however, Q1 and Q2 are important question items because they are related to the time it takes to manage diabetes and receive health checkups. Recently, AshaRani et al. [36] reported that the advantages of telemedicine included saving time, convenience and cost, and the most satisfactory telemedicine service was booking appointments. The results of this study suggest that patients expect improved access to healthcare through the implementation of telemedicine. Therefore, the questionnaire should include question items regarding accessibility, such as waiting time, appointment booking system and healthcare costs, to appropriately assess changes in patient satisfaction. The most frequently used telemedicine-specific questionnaire is the Telehealth Usability Questionnaire, which includes the question items regarding time travelling to healthcare organisations and access to healthcare services [32]; however, no question item on costs was noted. Telemedicine-specific questionnaires cannot be used to assess satisfaction in patients with conventional face-to-face care. A new comprehensive questionnaire should be developed to accurately assess patient satisfaction with telemedicine and validly compare patient satisfaction between patients receiving telemedicine and face-to-face care.

Interestingly, compared with patients without diabetes, those with diabetes prefer face-to-face visits over telemedicine [36]. Furthermore, most (75.7%) patients with diabetes seem to be not ready for telemedicine compared with those without diabetes (44.4%) owing to the following disadvantages of telemedicine: (1) requirement of digital literacy (94.3%), (2) difficulty in building good interpersonal relationships between clinicians and patients (81.0%), (3) not being credible (64.2%) and (4) not helpful for patients' health conditions (62.3%) [36]. Diabetes is a chronic disease, which makes continuity of care crucial. Patients who had a good interpersonal relationship with primary care physicians and high continuity of care had reduced mortality (odds ratio [OR] = 0.59; 95% CI, 0.50–0.70) and a lower risk of hospitalisation (OR = 0.82; 95% CI, 0.75–0.90) in addition to achieving better diabetes control [37]. Patient-centred care and interpersonal behaviours by healthcare providers could improve diabetes patients' trust and engagement in their management and the healthcare system [38]. Patient satisfaction is built based on individual subjective perception [39]; thus, objective assessment and the elimination of confounding factors are difficult. Moreover, the most crucial factor for building patient satisfaction is the interpersonal relationship between each patient and the healthcare provider [40]; therefore, who provides care to the patient may have more impact than what the healthcare provider uses for patient care. However, all the included studies did not mention differences in healthcare providers between telemedicine and in-person groups. The interpersonal relationship between healthcare providers and patients should be considered to truly assess the effect of telemedicine on patient satisfaction in patients with diabetes. Furthermore, patients' social relationships with their families, peers and healthcare providers significantly impact diabetes management across the life span [41]. Therefore, patients with diabetes may value a face-to-face relationship in their self-management.

One of the significant barriers to the implementation of telemedicine is the lack of digital literacy [42]. Particularly, older adults with lower income who are not familiar with digital devices have been found to experience difficulty in using telemedicine [43,44]. A systematic review concluded that older adults were satisfied with telemedicine during the COVID-19 pandemic; however, technical difficulties concerning the telemedicine delivery system were major barriers [45]. The average age of participants in Izquierdo et al. [21] and Sood et al. [28] was >60 years old, which may have affected patient satisfaction with telemedicine. However, most of the participants in the included studies were relatively young (30–50 years old), and the effect of telemedicine on patient satisfaction in older patients with diabetes was unknown. Considering that ageing is rapidly progressing worldwide, further studies investigating the effect of telemedicine on patient experience in older patients with diabetes are warranted.

Information technology has achieved a remarkable breakthrough. However, the author recognises the vital need for further technological advancements in healthcare to provide effective and efficient treatment to the increasing number of older patients worldwide. For example, 5G networks will be able to transfer a significantly higher volume of data than now, allowing healthcare providers to perform more real teleconsultation and telesurgery [46]. Moreover, the Internet of Things technology will assist older adults living alone with maintaining or improving activities of daily life [47]. Such information technology advancement in healthcare ensures connecting older adults and their families with healthcare resources and may improve physical and mental well-being [48], which contributes to establishing an integrated healthcare system in ageing communities.

Furthermore, the author has mentioned the issue of the study design in the included studies. In principle, implementing double-blind RCTs with subjective endpoints, such as patient satisfaction, is impossible. Study participants can realise which group they were allocated and how they were treated. However, at least the outcome assessor should be blinded (single-blind), as in the study by Yaron et al. [23].

This systematic review had some limitations. First, it was conducted by a single author; hence, biases in study selection and study quality assessment may exist. A systematic review with meta-analysis should be performed in the future with the inclusion of an adequate number of RCTs. Second, all of the included studies were not designed to assess patient satisfaction as a primary outcome. Further studies investigating the effect of telemedicine on patient satisfaction as a primary outcome are needed.

In conclusion, patient satisfaction was high in patients receiving telemedicine; however, the difference in patient satisfaction between telemedicine and face-to-face care was not significant. Considerable heterogeneities between studies were noted, including age and telemedicine delivery tools. Moreover, the effect of telemedicine on patient satisfaction as a primary outcome in older patients who are not ready for telemedicine due to a lack of digital literacy was not examined. Telemedicine should be more studied and developed in anticipation of the next pandemic or coming superageing societies. Telemedicine that establishes good interpersonal relationships between patients and healthcare providers and increases patient satisfaction is a key tool to providing high-quality healthcare to patients with diabetes in the 21st century.

Supplementary Materials: The following supporting information can be downloaded at: https://www.mdpi.com/article/10.3390/healthcare10091677/s1, PRISMA 2020 checklist.

Funding: This research received no external funding.

Institutional Review Board Statement: Not applicable.

Informed Consent Statement: Not applicable.

Data Availability Statement: The data that support the findings of this study are available from the corresponding author upon reasonable request.

Conflicts of Interest: The author declares no conflict of interest.

References

1. Kleinrock, L. History of the Internet and its flexible future. *IEEE Wirel. Commun.* **2008**, *15*, 8–18. [CrossRef]
2. Holroyd-Leduc, J.M.; Lorenzetti, D.; Straus, S.E.; Sykes, L.; Quan, H. The impact of the electronic medical record on structure, process, and outcomes within primary care: A systematic review of the evidence. *J. Am. Med. Inform. Assoc.* **2011**, *18*, 732–737. [CrossRef] [PubMed]
3. Ristevski, B.; Chen, M. Big Data Analytics in Medicine and Healthcare. *J. Integr. Bioinform.* **2018**, *15*, 20170030. [CrossRef] [PubMed]
4. Yu, K.H.; Beam, A.L.; Kohane, I.S. Artificial intelligence in healthcare. *Nat. Biomed. Eng.* **2018**, *2*, 719–731. [CrossRef] [PubMed]
5. Zhang, B. Expert Consensus on Telemedicine Management of Diabetes (2020 Edition). *Int. J. Endocrinol.* **2021**, *2021*, 6643491. [CrossRef]
6. Hangaard, S.; Laursen, S.H.; Andersen, J.D.; Kronborg, T.; Vestergaard, P.; Hejlesen, O.; Udsen, F.W. The Effectiveness of Telemedicine Solutions for the Management of Type 2 Diabetes: A Systematic Review, Meta-Analysis, and Meta-Regression. *J. Diabetes Sci. Technol.* **2021**, *26*, 19322968211064633. [CrossRef]
7. Lee, S.W.H.; Ooi, L.; Lai, Y.K. Telemedicine for the Management of Glycemic Control and Clinical Outcomes of Type 1 Diabetes Mellitus: A Systematic Review and Meta-Analysis of Randomized Controlled Studies. *Front. Pharmacol.* **2017**, *8*, 330. [CrossRef]
8. Lee, J.Y.; Lee, S.W.H. Telemedicine Cost-Effectiveness for Diabetes Management: A Systematic Review. *Diabetes Technol. Ther.* **2018**, *20*, 492–500. [CrossRef]
9. De Simone, S.; Franco, M.; Servillo, G.; Vargas, M. Implementations and strategies of telehealth during COVID-19 outbreak: A systematic review. *BMC Health Serv. Res.* **2022**, *22*, 833. [CrossRef]
10. Pogorzelska, K.; Chlabicz, S. Patient Satisfaction with Telemedicine during the COVID-19 Pandemic-A Systematic Review. *Int. J. Environ. Res. Public Health* **2022**, *19*, 6113. [CrossRef]
11. Zhang, W.; Cheng, B.; Zhu, W.; Huang, X.; Shen, C. Effect of Telemedicine on Quality of Care in Patients with Coexisting Hypertension and Diabetes: A Systematic Review and Meta-Analysis. *Telemed. J. e-Health* **2021**, *27*, 603–614. [CrossRef]
12. Flodgren, G.; Rachas, A.; Farmer, A.J.; Inzitari, M.; Shepperd, S. Interactive telemedicine: Effects on professional practice and health care outcomes. *Cochrane Database Syst. Rev.* **2015**, *2016*, CD002098. [CrossRef] [PubMed]
13. Kruse, C.S.; Krowski, N.; Rodriguez, B.; Tran, L.; Vela, J.; Brooks, M. Telehealth and patient satisfaction: A systematic review and narrative analysis. *BMJ Open* **2017**, *7*, e016242. [CrossRef]
14. Pascoe, G.C. Patient satisfaction in primary health care: A literature review and analysis. *Eval. Program Plan.* **1983**, *6*, 185–210. [CrossRef]
15. Sitzia, J.; Wood, N. Patient satisfaction: A review of issues and concepts. *Soc. Sci. Med.* **1997**, *45*, 1829–1843. [CrossRef]
16. Page, M.J.; McKenzie, J.E.; Bossuyt, P.M.; Boutron, I.; Hoffmann, T.C.; Mulrow, C.D.; Shamseer, L.; Tetzlaff, J.M.; Akl, E.A.; Brennan, S.E.; et al. The PRISMA 2020 statement: An updated guideline for reporting systematic reviews. *BMJ* **2021**, *372*, n71. [CrossRef] [PubMed]
17. National Institute of Health National; Institute of Biomedical Imaging and Bioengineering. Telehealth. Available online: https://www.nibib.nih.gov/science-education/science-topics/telehealth (accessed on 21 August 2022).
18. Sood, S.; Mbarika, V.; Jugoo, S.; Dookhy, R.; Doarn, C.; Prakash, N.; Merrell, R.C. What is telemedicine? A collection of 104 peer-reviewed perspectives and theoretical underpinnings. *Telemed. J. e-Health* **2007**, *13*, 573–590. [CrossRef] [PubMed]
19. Sterne, J.A.C.; Savović, J.; Page, M.J.; Elbers, R.G.; Blencowe, N.S.; Boutron, I.; Cates, C.J.; Cheng, H.Y.; Corbett, M.S.; Eldridge, S.M.; et al. RoB 2: A revised tool for assessing risk of bias in randomised trials. *BMJ* **2019**, *366*, l4898. [CrossRef]
20. Riskofbias.Info. Available online: https://www.riskofbias.info/ (accessed on 7 July 2022).
21. Izquierdo, R.E.; Knudson, P.E.; Meyer, S.; Kearns, J.; Ploutz-Snyder, R.; Weinstock, R.S. A comparison of diabetes education administered through telemedicine versus in person. *Diabetes Care* **2003**, *26*, 1002–1007. [CrossRef]
22. Institute of Medicine (US) Committee on Evaluating Clinical Applications of Telemedicine. *Telemedicine: A Guide to Assessing Telecommunications in Health Care*; Field, M.J., Ed.; National Academies Press: Washington, DC, USA, 1996.
23. Yaron, M.; Sher, B.; Sorek, D.; Shomer, M.; Levek, N.; Schiller, T.; Gaspar, M.; Ben-David, R.F.; Mazor-Aronovitch, K.; Tish, E.; et al. A randomized controlled trial comparing a telemedicine therapeutic intervention with routine care in adults with type 1 diabetes mellitus treated by insulin pumps. *Acta Diabetol.* **2019**, *56*, 667–673. [CrossRef]
24. Cho, J.H.; Kim, H.-S.; Yoo, S.H.; Jung, C.H.; Lee, W.J.; Park, C.Y.; Yang, H.K.; Park, J.Y.; Park, S.W.; Yoon, K.H. An Internet-based health gateway device for interactive communication and automatic data uploading: Clinical efficacy for type 2 diabetes in a multi-centre trial. *J. Telemed. Telecare* **2016**, *23*, 595–604. [CrossRef] [PubMed]
25. Kirwan, M.; Vandelanotte, C.; Fenning, A.; Duncan, M.J. Diabetes self-management smartphone application for adults with type 1 diabetes: Randomized controlled trial. *J. Med. Internet Res.* **2013**, *15*, e235. [CrossRef]
26. Mulvaney, S.A.; Ritterband, L.M.; Bosslet, L. Mobile intervention design in diabetes: Review and recommendations. *Curr. Diabetes Rep.* **2011**, *11*, 486–493. [CrossRef] [PubMed]

27. de Adana, M.S.R.; Alhambra-Expósito, M.R.; Muñoz-Garach, A.; Gonzalez-Molero, I.; Colomo, N.; Torres-Barea, I.; Aguilar-Diosdado, M.; Carral, F.; Serrano, M.; Martínez-Brocca, M.A.; et al. Diabetes Group of SAEDYN (Andalusian Society of Endocrinology, Diabetes, and Nutrition). Randomized Study to Evaluate the Impact of Telemedicine Care in Patients With Type 1 Diabetes With Multiple Doses of Insulin and Suboptimal HbA1c in Andalusia (Spain): PLATEDIAN Study. *Diabetes Care* **2019**, *43*, 337–342. [CrossRef]
28. Sood, A.; A Watts, S.; Johnson, J.K.; Hirth, S.; Aron, D.C. Telemedicine consultation for patients with diabetes mellitus: A cluster randomised controlled trial. *J. Telemed. Telecare* **2017**, *24*, 385–391. [CrossRef]
29. Dananjayan, S.; Raj, G.M. 5G in healthcare: How fast will be the transformation? *Ir. J. Med. Sci.* **2020**, *190*, 497–501. [CrossRef]
30. Rubin, H.R.; Gandek, B.; Rogers, W.H.; Kosinski, M.; McHorney, C.A.; Ware, J.E., Jr. Patients' ratings of outpatient visits in different practice settings. Results from the Medical Outcomes Study. *JAMA* **1993**, *270*, 835–840. [CrossRef]
31. Bayley, K.B.; London, M.R.; Grunkemeier, G.L.; Lansky, D.J. Measuring the success of treatment in patient terms. *Med. Care* **1995**, *33* (Suppl. 4), AS226–AS235.
32. Hajesmaeel-Gohari, S.; Bahaadinbeigy, K. The most used questionnaires for evaluating telemedicine services. *BMC Med. Inform. Decis. Mak.* **2021**, *21*, 36. [CrossRef]
33. Saisho, Y. Use of Diabetes Treatment Satisfaction Questionnaire in Diabetes Care: Importance of Patient-Reported Outcomes. *Int. J. Environ. Res. Public Health* **2018**, *15*, 947. [CrossRef]
34. Bradley, C. The diabetes treatment satisfaction questionnaire: DTSQ. In *Handbook of Psychology and Diabetes: A Guide to Psychological Measurement in Diabetes Research and Practice*; Harwood Academic Publishers: Chur, Switzerland, 1994; pp. 111–132.
35. The DCCT Research Group. Reliability and validity of a diabetes quality-of-life measure for the diabetes control and complications trial (DCCT). *Diabetes Care* **1988**, *11*, 725–732. [CrossRef] [PubMed]
36. AshaRani, P.; Hua, L.J.; Roystonn, K.; Kumar, F.D.S.; Peizhi, W.; Jie, S.Y.; Shafie, S.; Chang, S.; Jeyagurunathan, A.; Yiang, C.B.; et al. Readiness and Acceptance of eHealth Services for Diabetes Care in the General Population: Cross-sectional Study. *J. Med. Internet Res.* **2021**, *23*, e26881. [CrossRef]
37. Lustman, A.; Comaneshter, D.; Vinker, S. Interpersonal continuity of care and type two diabetes. *Prim. Care Diabetes* **2016**, *10*, 165–170. [CrossRef] [PubMed]
38. Ciechanowski, P.; Katon, W.J. The interpersonal experience of health care through the eyes of patients with diabetes. *Soc. Sci. Med.* **2006**, *63*, 3067–3079. [CrossRef] [PubMed]
39. Crow, R.; Gage, H.; Hampson, S.; Hart, J.; Kimber, A.; Storey, L.; Thomas, H. The measurement of satisfaction with healthcare: Implications for practice from a systematic review of the literature. *Health Technol. Assess.* **2002**, *6*, 1–244. [CrossRef]
40. Gill, L.; White, L. A critical review of patient satisfaction. *Leadersh. Health Serv.* **2009**, *22*, 8–19. [CrossRef]
41. Wiebe, D.J.; Helgeson, V.; Berg, C.A. The social context of managing diabetes across the life span. *Am. Psychol.* **2016**, *71*, 526–538. [CrossRef]
42. Kruse, C.S.; Karem, P.; Shifflett, K.; Vegi, L.; Ravi, K.; Brooks, M. Evaluating barriers to adopting telemedicine worldwide: A systematic review. *J. Telemed. Telecare* **2018**, *24*, 4–12. [CrossRef]
43. Kuang, W.; Zeng, G.; Nie, Y.; Cai, Y.; Li, J.; Wan, Y.; Qiu, P. Equity in telemedicine for older adults during the COVID-19 pandemic. *Int. Health* **2021**, *14*, 329–331. [CrossRef]
44. Choi, N.G.; DiNitto, D.M.; Marti, C.N.; Choi, B.Y. Telehealth Use Among Older Adults During COVID-19: Associations with Sociodemographic and Health Characteristics, Technology Device Ownership, and Technology Learning. *J. Appl. Gerontol.* **2021**, *41*, 600–609. [CrossRef]
45. Alsabeeha, N.H.; Atieh, M.A.; Balakrishnan, M.S. Older Adults' Satisfaction with Telemedicine During the COVID-19 Pandemic: A Systematic Review. *Telemed. J. e-Health* **2022**, Available online: https://www.liebertpub.com/doi/10.1089/tmj.2022.0045 (accessed on 1 March 2022). [CrossRef]
46. Ullah, H.; Nair, N.G.; Moore, A.; Nugent, C.; Muschamp, P.; Cuevas, M. 5G communication: An overview of vehicle-to-everything, drones, and healthcare use-cases. *IEEE Access* **2019**, *7*, 37251–37268. [CrossRef]
47. Baig, M.M.; Afifi, S.; GholamHosseini, H.; Mirza, F. A Systematic Review of Wearable Sensors and IoT-Based Monitoring Applications for Older Adults—A Focus on Ageing Population and Independent Living. *J. Med. Syst.* **2019**, *43*, 233. [CrossRef] [PubMed]
48. Sen, K.; Prybutok, G.; Prybutok, V. The use of digital technology for social wellbeing reduces social isolation in older adults: A systematic review. *SSM Popul. Health* **2021**, *17*, 101020. [CrossRef] [PubMed]

MDPI AG
Grosspeteranlage 5
4052 Basel
Switzerland
Tel.: +41 61 683 77 34

Healthcare Editorial Office
E-mail: healthcare@mdpi.com
www.mdpi.com/journal/healthcare

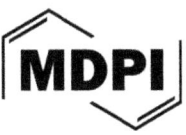

Disclaimer/Publisher's Note: The statements, opinions and data contained in all publications are solely those of the individual author(s) and contributor(s) and not of MDPI and/or the editor(s). MDPI and/or the editor(s) disclaim responsibility for any injury to people or property resulting from any ideas, methods, instructions or products referred to in the content.